Nurses' Aids Series

PERSONAL AND COMMUNITY HEALTH

Nurses' Aids Series

Personal and Community Health

Sheila M. Jackson
SRN, SCM, BTA, RNT
Inspector of Training Schools for the
General Nursing Council for England and Wales
Formerly Nurse Tutor, Queen Elizabeth School of Nursing,
Birmingham, and St Charles' Hospital, London

and

Susan Lane
SRN, RSCN, HV
Health Visitor, Kensington, Chelsea and Westminster A.H.A.

BAILLIÈRE TINDALL ✤ LONDON

BAILLIÈRE TINDALL
7 & 8 Henrietta Street, London WC2E 8QE

Cassell & Collier Macmillan Publishers Ltd., London
35 Red Lion Square, London WC1R 4SG
Sydney, Auckland, Toronto, Johannesburg

The Macmillan Publishing Company Inc.
New York

First published as *Aids to Hygiene for Nurses* by E. Funnell,
1938
Fifth Edition 1956 (Reprinted 5 times)
Personal and Community Health by W. L. Huntly, 1964
Second Edition 1969
Personal and Community Health by S. M. Jackson and
S. Lane, 1975

Limp Edition ISBN 0 7020 0576 2

Printed by Cox & Wyman Ltd,
London, Fakenham and Reading

Contents

Preface

'The nurse has an important part to play as a health teacher and must have a knowledge of the factors in the environment which give rise to ill health since she will be called upon to advise patients and their relatives on how to care for themselves and their family in a way which will promote a state of physical and mental well-being.'

This quotation from the preface to the 1969 syllabus of subjects for examination for the certificate of general nursing, published by the General Nursing Council for England and Wales, has been the key to what we have tried to achieve in the third approach to this subject, now in two distinct parts. The first section shows the measures which an individual should take to maintain his own health or which should be taken for him if he is too young; the second section indicates the main responsibilities which the community must undertake to achieve optimum health in the population as a whole.

The chapters on health education include the reasons behind the various hygienic practices described and mention the difficulties and dangers which arise if such practices are neglected. They also discuss briefly the more common departures from healthy living which present problems today and in the prevention of which improved health education is an important factor.

Stress has been laid throughout the book on mental health and the contributions which can be made to its establishment and maintenance. The health and standards of hygiene of the United Kingdom are improving all the time but perhaps insufficient attention has been paid to the psychological aspects without which physiological health has no meaning.

An outline is given of the functions of the primary health care team and of the services available to help in the restoration of health following illness or injury. Many of the social services which have an indirect effect on the health of the individual are also mentioned.

It is hoped that the provision of a comprehensive index will enable information to be found easily and that the Background Readings, arranged to follow the sequence of this book, will be useful to those who enjoy reading more widely about a subject of particular interest.

We would like to thank our friends and relations who have borne with us so patiently while this book has been in preparation and our professional colleagues throughout the country who have added their contributions by giving us the benefit of their knowledge and opinions—in many cases unwittingly! Special thanks are due to Wendy Chamberlain who has typed the entire manuscript for us with unfailing punctuality and good humour and to the publishers who have as usual given us their continued support and help.

June 1975   S. M. JACKSON
                                               S. LANE

ACKNOWLEDGEMENTS

We wish to acknowledge our gratitude for permission granted by the General Nursing Council for England and Wales to quote from the syllabus and to those who have provided us with the following: Figs. 4, 5 and 6 – reproduced from 'New Baby' by permission of the publishers B. Edsall & Co. Limited; Fig. 9 – Redemptorist Publications; Figs. 16 and 17 – Sneddon & Church, *Practical Dermatology*, 2nd ed. London, Edward Arnold Ltd. 1971; Fig. 24 – Department of the Environment; Fig. 25 – Dr Claude Nicol; Fig. 28 – J. Carter, Upper Ladbroke School, London W.10; Fig. 34 – Electrolux Ltd, Hoover Ltd, and Sydney Flavel & Co. Ltd; Fig. 35 – Trevor Poyser; Fig. 38 – Shell-Mex and B.P. Ltd; Fig. 39 – Marks & Spencer Ltd; and Fig. 40 – Department of Management Studies, North London Polytechnic.

PERSONAL HEALTH

The Expectant Mother

Antenatal Care

The future health of every individual begins before birth and much can be done in the nine months following conception to ensure that everything possible is done to secure a good start in life for the new baby.

Aims of Antenatal Care

The aims of antenatal care are:

1. To maintain and improve the health of the mother.
2. To prevent obstetric abnormality and to diagnose and treat unavoidable complications as early as possible.
3. To promote full development of the fetus so that a healthy baby is delivered.
4. To teach the mother about pregnancy and childbirth and how to care for her baby when it is born.

The fact that these aims are being achieved is shown by the trends in mortality rates for mothers and babies in recent years. Thirty years ago four or five women died in pregnancy or during childbirth for every thousand births; now the figure is less than one for every five thousand births. Similarly about sixty babies died as a direct result of birth processes for every one thousand born alive; now the figure is about twenty-five for every thousand (see also Chapter 13).

Routine Antenatal Care

A woman is likely to suspect she is pregnant when she misses a menstrual period. Additionally, about six weeks after the onset of the last normal period she may experience feelings of nausea. Her first move is likely to be a visit to her own doctor in order that the pregnancy may be confirmed, after which plans may be made for her subsequent care. It may be arranged that antenatal supervision will be carried out by her own doctor, particularly if he has a special interest in obstetrics, or the woman may attend an antenatal clinic held in a local health centre and conducted by local midwives.

Increasing numbers of women are having their babies in hospital and in this case they will attend the hospital antenatal clinic for at least some part of their care and possibly for all of it. Where home conditions and the woman's previous obstetric history are satisfactory and where the woman herself is anxious to have the baby at home this can be arranged and the home will then be visited by the midwife who will attend the delivery. Advice will be given about the domestic arrangements and the conditions in which the baby will be born.

At the first visit to the antenatal clinic a full record of her previous medical and obstetric history will be made and she will be asked about the duration and regularity of her usual menstrual cycle. If this is irregular it will be difficult to give an accurate forecast of the date of delivery. The average duration of pregnancy in humans is 40 weeks or 266 days from the date of conception. Calculations are usually based on the date of the first day of the last normal menstrual period, since this is frequently an easier date to determine than the actual date of conception. A quick way of calculating the date of delivery is to add seven days to the date of the first day of the last normal menstrual period and then to subtract three months from this date. If the last menstrual period starts on December 4th, 1984, add on seven days (December 11th) and subtract three months (September). The baby would be expected about September 11th, 1985, though it must be made clear that this date is only approximate and it is not unusual or abnormal for a baby to arrive up to a fortnight before or after the expected date of delivery.

A full medical examination is carried out by the doctor at the first visit to the clinic to assess the general health of the woman and to establish a base line against which any changes during pregnancy can be compared. Particular attention is paid to the blood pressure and to examination of the urine for sugar and albumen, as an increase in these levels later in pregnancy may indicate the onset of toxaemia of pregnancy.

Other investigations which are carried out at the beginning of pregnancy include a chest X-ray and investigation of the blood. It is important to know the blood group and whether the Rhesus factor is present. If it is not, the blood is examined for the presence of rhesus antibodies which may act adversely on the blood of the fetus. Tests are also carried out to exclude syphilis and gonorrhoea.

If all goes well subsequent antenatal visits will be arranged at four-weekly intervals until the twenty-eighth week of pregnancy, three-weekly intervals until the thirty-fourth week, fortnightly until the thirty-sixth week and weekly thereafter. At each of these visits the woman is questioned about her general health and her urine is tested and her blood pressure measured. Her abdomen will be palpated to ascertain the size of the uterus and the lie of the fetus, and her hands and feet will be examined for oedema, which may also herald the onset of toxaemia of pregnancy. If there is some doubt about clinical signs an X-ray may be taken but this is only done during pregnancy if it is essential, as there is some evidence that fetal exposure to X-rays in utero may increase the risk of malignant disease in childhood.

Advice during Pregnancy

During her attendance at antenatal clinics the woman will receive advice on the part that she can play in producing a healthy baby. This advice may come in the form of group discussions and talks which she may attend, it may be gained from leaflets which are freely available at the clinic, or from individual discussions with the health visitor or midwife. Most women are particularly receptive to advice during pregnancy and it is a good opportunity to teach them some principles of general health care as well as those points specifically relevant to pregnancy.

A woman should eat the *foods* she is normally accustomed to. It is no time to attempt radical changes in eating habits and the advice is unlikely to be taken if it is given. She should however be encouraged to eat plenty of meat, fish, eggs and dairy products as they supply the protein and calcium needed for normal fetal development. One pint of milk a day should be taken in drinks and in cooking, and vitamin supplements, available from the antenatal clinic, should be taken regularly. Fresh fruit and vegetables and an adequate intake of fluids are important in the prevention of constipation which is sometimes a problem in pregnancy. Excessive amounts of carbohydrate should be avoided as this causes weight gain which is thought to predispose to toxaemia. The old adage of 'eating for two' should be ignored, but there is evidence to suggest that a daily intake of less than 2500 calories and less than 20 per cent protein may be a cause of increased risk of infant mortality (see also Chapter 5).

Diet is important in order that there is not too much *weight gain* during pregnancy. A woman should not gain more than 10 kg (22 lb) during the entire nine-month period and after the first three months about 1·5 kg (3½ lb) each month should be the aim. The weight will be recorded at each clinic visit as excessive gain may be due to the onset of toxaemia, and is thought actually to increase the incidence of this condition.

The tendency to *tooth decay* is not lessened during pregnancy and regular visits to the dentist are important. In Britain visits are free during pregnancy and for one year after. It was considered at one time that if the mother's intake of calcium was insufficient during pregnancy the calcium needed for the development of the bones of the fetus was obtained from the teeth and bones of the mother, but it is now established that under these circumstances it is the mother's bones which supply any deficiency in calcium and not her teeth. Regular thorough brushing of the teeth in the correct way and eating correct foods such as celery and apples are helpful in maintaining healthy teeth (see also Chapter 5).

Some women find *morning sickness* a great problem in early pregnancy and it is very distressing to wake up each morning feeling nauseated whether or not there is actual vomiting. A woman should be advised to go to bed sufficiently early that she does not have to get up immediately she wakes. A dry biscuit, with a drink of whatever can be tolerated, seems to help some people, while in others a spoonful of sugar or honey is effective. In either case to continue lying down for a while, then to get up slowly and to eat a good breakfast will help the nausea to pass off.

Plenty of *rest* is important during pregnancy. In the early months it is sufficient to ensure a good night's sleep. In the later months it is advisable to have a rest with the feet up after lunch each day in addition to a good night's rest.

A normal amount of *exercise* is essential in the maintenance of health and should be continued during pregnancy. Tennis, golf, walking or swimming, in the fresh air whenever possible, are beneficial for a healthy woman but more violent sports such as riding, diving and ski-ing are probably best avoided.

If a woman has a job it is quite in order to remain at *work*, as long as she is well, until at least three months before the date of delivery and in many cases for even longer. However, as mentioned above, she should not become overtired and it may be necessary to find a job which does not entail excessive amounts of standing (see 'Maternity Allowance' p. 12).

Clothes should be comfortable and not too tight. It is advisable for the woman to buy a well-fitting brassière to support the breasts which will begin to enlarge quite early in pregnancy. Unless the abdominal muscles are very slack there is no necessity to wear a girdle or corset. High-heeled shoes should be avoided because they tend to throw the body off balance (see Fig. 1), though if a woman has always worn fairly high heels she should not make a sudden change to flat shoes. A heel of about $1\frac{1}{2}$ to 2 inches is probably best.

Personal hygiene is as important during pregnancy as at any other time. A daily bath, or wash all over, is refreshing and cleansing and helps to keep the skin in good condition. Special attention should be paid to the breasts and it will be part of the duty of the midwife to give advice if the nipples are retracted or liable to crack.

Pregnant women should be encouraged to give up, or at least to reduce, *smoking*. There is evidence to show that there is an increased risk of abortion or of premature labour in the heavy smoker and that the babies of these women are smaller than the babies of non-smokers. It is thought that the reasons for this may be to do with the increase in the level of carbon monoxide in maternal and fetal circulation which leads to a corresponding impairment of oxygenation, and also that the

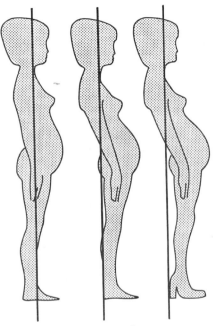

1. The effect of high heels on posture during pregnancy; the weight is thrown even farther back putting added strain on the curve of the spine and increasing the likelihood of loss of balance.

vasoconstrictor effect of nicotine will affect the placental vessels (see Chapter 6).

Intercourse may be safely enjoyed during pregnancy unless there is a history of previous miscarriages. It is best avoided in the latter months of pregnancy.

Those *drugs* which are not specifically prescribed by a

doctor are best avoided during pregnancy. Only a doctor can be sure which drugs have been adequately tested and have been proven safe to be taken during pregnancy. Drugs which a woman may take quite safely when she is not pregnant may affect the fetus adversely because the adult dose will be far too much for the incompletely developed fetal liver to detoxicate. Some drugs have a very specific effect on the developing fetus. The best-known example is thalidomide which, if taken between the 27th and 40th days after conception, causes incorrect development of the arms and legs of the fetus.

Some *infections* have a specific effect on the developing fetus, the best known being rubella (German measles). If a woman is infected with this virus during the first three months of pregnancy the baby may be born with congenital cataracts, the ears and heart may also be affected. Preventive immunization of girls may be about the age of twelve to prevent this tragedy. A pregnant woman who comes in contact with a case of rubella during the significant months and who has not been protected against the infection should notify her doctor and may be given passive protection. Another infection which may affect the fetus is syphilis and this must be adequately treated during pregnancy if the baby is to be born healthy.

Of course there is little that can be done to control the *emotions* but there is evidence to show that the emotional state of the woman can affect the fetus, so anything which helps to bring peace of mind and happiness will be beneficial.

All the measures to create good health mentioned above will help, particularly because the mother will feel she is doing all she can to give the baby a good start in life. A woman who is pregnant needs support from her husband and family and while there is no need for her to be treated as an invalid they should show interest in her progress and give her encouragement to fulfil all the measures for safeguarding her own health. They may also provide some diversion and help her to enjoy the time before the new baby arrives.

Preparation for Parenthood

During pregnancy a woman should attend classes in mother-craft during which she is able to learn all she needs to know about the care of a new baby, an aspect of parenthood which may unnerve some young mothers unless they are adequately prepared. Husbands also should be encouraged to attend these classes so that they can learn alongside their wives and be able to help out, both practically and emotionally, when necessary.

Relaxation classes, run by a health visitor or midwife, are also available, and in addition to learning the valuable art of relaxing the mother also learns what to expect of her pregnancy and labour. This knowledge helps to dispel fear and to improve confidence and may make the difference between enjoying pregnancy, or regarding it as a nuisance to be got through as quickly as possible.

In Britain classes organized by the National Childbirth Trust are also available. The Trust is a national organization which exists to educate people for parenthood and to train expectant mothers to develop a positive attitude to birth. The Trust employs trained teachers who give antenatal preparation classes. These are concerned with teaching mothers the ability to keep at rest all muscles not directly concerned with labour, and also teaching a pattern of 'conscious controlled breathing'. This technique enables the mother to feel actively involved in controlling her own labour and in the subsequent birth of her child.

Maternity Services in Britain

Providing the necessary contributions have been paid a *maternity allowance* is paid to every expectant mother for eleven weeks before the birth and seven weeks afterwards and is designed to encourage the working woman to give up her job during the later stages of pregnancy and the important weeks after delivery. A *maternity grant* is a lump sum payment for each child alive twelve hours after birth. The amounts of these allowances change frequently and the current amount payable can be ascertained from the local Social Security office, the address of which can be obtained from the Post Office.

A pregnant woman can obtain any item ordered by a doctor on a *prescription form* from the chemist free of charge and she is also entitled to *free dental treatment* for the duration of the pregnancy and for one year thereafter. Certain *welfare foods* are available free or at a reduced charge to expectant and nursing mothers. During her pregnancy a woman who has two or more children under school age can have seven pints of milk free each week or a packet of National Dried Milk if she prefers it. She can also obtain tablets containing Vitamins A, C and D to supplement her diet to a total of two packets every thirteen weeks.

If it has been decided that the baby will be born at home, arrangements will be made for a *midwife* to attend the mother and either the midwife or the general practitioner obstetrician will deliver the baby. It is necessary to arrange for help in the home during labour and the lying-in period and often a neighbour or relative is willing to help in this way. If there is no-one suitable, application may be made for a *home help*. This service, which is the responsibility of the local authority, will provide a worker who will run the home during the required period, doing shopping, cooking and housework and looking after other children as necessary. A charge will be made for this service, though financial help may be given if the full cost cannot be met.

Before the time of the delivery a *maternity pack* will be delivered to the house. This contains necessities for the delivery and should be left unopened until the midwife arrives.

A further service which is available when needed is the *emergency obstetric service*, usually known as the 'Flying Squad'. If there is a sudden emergency during a domiciliary delivery the midwife or doctor can summon help and the team, usually consisting of an experienced obstetrician and one or two midwives, will arrive with a specially equipped ambulance. Following immediate treatment the mother and baby can then be transferred to the hospital for further care.

Following the birth the midwife will attend mother and baby once or twice daily for seven to ten days, extending to fourteen days if necessary. After this time the care of the family becomes the responsibility of the health visitor.

Some women are admitted to hospital for the delivery and if all goes well are transferred to their own homes after 48 hours. The midwife carries out the care of mother and baby as she would if the delivery had taken place at home. This scheme known as 'planned early discharge' works well in many areas and in some the domiciliary midwife accompanies the mother to hospital and delivers her there, just as she would at home.

Where there are older children in the family arrangements must be made for their care and supervision while the mother is unable to look after them. If there is no relative to care for them or a home help cannot be arranged it is possible for them to be taken into care for a short time.

Postnatal Care

Many mothers experience mixed feelings after the birth of a baby, particularly when they are first left to care for it. In the beginning there is the natural delight and pride in her achievement and the hopeful expectations for the future. Later it is common to experience great apprehension as she becomes more aware of the tremendous responsibility and this is often followed by anticlimax as she becomes aware of physical tiredness. A great deal of support is needed at this time and should be given by family and friends as well as by the health visitor.

The mother should continue the nourishing diet and vitamin supplements she was taking during pregnancy and this is particularly important if the baby is being breast fed. She should try to avoid heavy work and prolonged standing and the daily rest should be continued if possible. She should also continue the exercises she has been shown in order to tone up the muscles both internally and externally and, incidentally, to help in regaining her figure. Intercourse should be avoided for at least six weeks and it is at this point that the mother may be most receptive to advice regarding contraception so that she can avoid an unplanned pregnancy.

Six weeks after delivery a visit should be paid to the clinic for a postnatal examination to ensure that all is well and that involution is progressing normally.

Family Planning

The facts regarding contraception must be known and understood so that they can be discussed freely and advice can be given without ethical or religious bias. Individual advice on family planning can be obtained at any one of numerous clinics up and down the country. Information about local clinics can be obtained from the Citizens' Advice Bureau, local council offices or the health visitor.

The only method of contraception approved by the Roman Catholic Church at the present time is the *safe period*. Intercourse must occur only when there is no ovum to be fertilized. Ovulation occurs fourteen days before the menstrual period so if the cycle is regular the date of ovulation can be calculated. Spermatozoa live in the female genital tract for about five days so it would be unwise to have intercourse for five days before and for five days after ovulation. This method can only be successful if the cycle is regular and if there is total abstention from intercourse for some part of every cycle. For these reasons it cannot be considered satisfactory or completely reliable.

Coitus interruptus is also unreliable as a method of contraception. The male organ is withdrawn from the vagina before ejaculation of any spermatozoa. This may cause suffering and frustration and is not conducive to satisfying relationships between husband and wife. There is some evidence to show that it causes backache and dysmenorrhoea through congestion of the pelvic organs if it is continued.

A far more reliable method is for the woman to take a *contraceptive drug*. These contain hormones which act on the anterior lobe of the hypophysis and inhibit ovulation and act on the endometrium, altering it so that it is not ready to receive a fertilized ovum. The pill is taken from the fifth day of the cycle for twenty-one days and then is discontinued for seven days, during which bleeding will occur.

For women who have already had a baby, and in some cases for those who have not, an *intrauterine contraceptive device* (IUCD or IUD) may be inserted (see Fig. 2). These are made of plastic or stainless steel and are inserted into the uterus and left there. There are several different types and they probably work by preventing implantation. They are not entirely without complications and are probably most useful where other methods cannot be used.

An *occlusive diaphragm* or Dutch cap is a shaped piece of latex attached to a compressible spring rather like a ring pessary (see Fig. 3). It is placed in position between cervix and vagina and acts as a mechanical barrier to the spermatozoa. It should be used in conjunction with spermicidal cream and should not be removed for at least eight hours after intercourse. It is a safe method if used correctly.

Spermicidal pessaries and cream are not safe if used alone.

A *condom* is a latex sheath which is fitted over the penis before intercourse. It is reliable if it is intact and is fitted soon enough.

Surgical sterilization may be carried out for either men or women. *Vasectomy* is a comparatively minor operation for men involving division of the deferent duct. For women, tying or *division of the uterine tubes* involves rather more major surgery.

Genetic Counselling

If parents have had the misfortune to have a baby who has some congenital abnormality or inherited constitutional defect, or if one or other parent suffers from a condition which may be passed on to a child they may be advised by their doctor to seek advice from a geneticist. The genetic counsellor will make a diagnosis based on full clinical examination and whatever laboratory investigations seem necessary. The availability and value of any possible treatment will be discussed and the prognosis indicated. Finally frank discussion

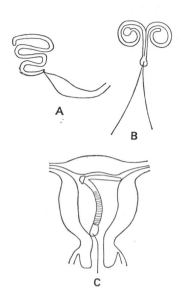

2. Some intrauterine contraceptive devices, A, Lippes loop; B, Saf-t-coil; C, Gravigard in uterus.

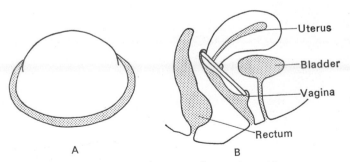

3. A, Diaphragm (Dutch cap); B, Diaphragm in position.

with the parents will help to relieve any feelings of guilt they may have and will help them in making a decision. Advice can be given about the likelihood of a condition being transmitted to a child or in cases of hermaphroditism guidance can be given as to whether it would be best to bring the child up as a girl or a boy.

2

The Infant

Notification and Registration of Birth

Within 36 hours of delivery the midwife or doctor in attendance must *notify* the Medical Officer of Health of the birth. This notification has been compulsory in Britain since 1915. It is the duty of one of the parents to *register* the birth with the local registrar of births, deaths and marriages within 42 days of delivery, whether it was a live birth or a stillbirth.

Hygiene

It is customary to bath a small baby each day, preferably at the same time so that a routine is established. Many mothers find that just before the 10 a.m. feed is suitable as the morning rush is over and they feel more able to spend time with the baby. There is no reason why some other time of day should not be chosen to suit the convenience of the mother and family and to bath the baby just before the 6 p.m. feed is found to be satisfactory in some families. It is important that the room in which the baby is bathed is warm and free from draughts and that everything is prepared so that the risk of chilling the baby is reduced. The correct method of holding a baby in a bath is shown in Fig. 4. When bathing a boy it is important to remember that the foreskin is normally adherent after birth and cannot be retracted without causing bleeding so no attempts should be made to do this. Separation will occur naturally after a few weeks or months.

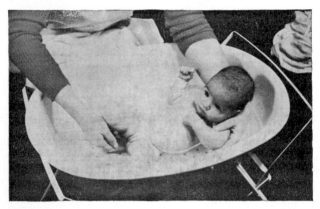

4. The correct method of holding the baby in the bath (B. Edsall & Co.).

Feeding

The small baby will require a feed every 3 to 4 hours, or he may be fed 'on demand' which in practice usually means that he will establish a routine of his own, similar to one which is imposed on him. It is important to remember that feeding time belongs to the baby and should be shared only with his mother or whoever is feeding him. He should be held closely and comfortably and attention should be focused on him while he sucks. It should not be a time when mother can hold a conversation with a friend, read a book, listen to a play or watch television. Breast feeding is of course the ideal way to feed a new baby (see Fig. 5). The milk contains exactly the right constituents for the baby, it is pure, clean and fresh, takes no time or trouble to prepare, costs nothing and is always ready wherever and whenever it is required. In addition it increases the baby's resistance to disease and

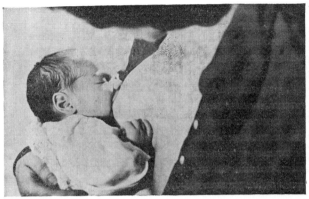

5. The correct method of holding the baby during breast feeding (B. Edsall & Co.).

helps in the formation of jaws and teeth while simultaneously there is a special bond between the breast-fed baby and his mother which no bottle feed can ever quite replace.

If the baby cannot be breast fed the artificial feeds available today enable a baby to thrive as well as a breast-fed baby provided he is cradled and comforted just as he would be if he were being breast fed (see Fig. 6). Extreme care must be taken in the preparation of the feeds so that amounts are measured accurately and the milk does not become contaminated. Supplementary vitamins in the form of vitamin A, C and D drops may be given and can be obtained at welfare clinics very cheaply.

The introduction of new foods usually begins about the

age of three months or when the baby weighs about 7 kg (15 lb). Very small quantities of puréed foods are offered starting with bland tastes and only gradually introducing more definite ones. The temptation to give too much cereal with added sugar should be resisted as it has been known

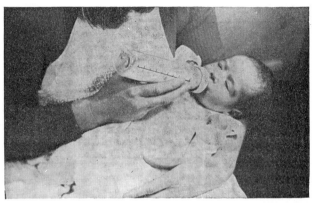

6. The correct method of holding the baby during bottle feeding (B. Edsall & Co.).

to cause colic in some babies and may cause obesity. Babies who are overweight at the age of six months are more likely to be overweight by the time they are five years than are normal children. Overnutrition in early life results in an increase in the number of fat cells in the body. Weight reduction later can only be due to reduction in the size of the cells as the number will remain constant.

Sleep

A new baby will sleep most of the 24 hours, waking only for feeding or if he is uncomfortable. He should be placed on one side in the cot or pram and should not have a pillow. The mattress should be soft and firm and have a protective cover over it and bedclothes should be light and warm. Cellular blankets are very suitable for babies' cots. Later when he becomes more active a sleeping bag may help to keep him warm until he goes to sleep. A baby who is clean, satisfied,

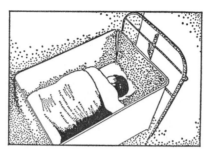

7. Baby securely settled in a cot.

comfortable and warm before he is put down to sleep should settle quickly and there should be no need for any undue hush or walking about on tiptoe. During the day if the weather is fine 2 to 3 hours spent in the fresh air will be beneficial, but a baby should not be put outside if the weather is foggy or bitterly cold. A cat-net should be put over the pram of a small baby.

Exercise

A certain time should be set aside each day when the baby is left free to exercise the limbs. He will also be encouraged to do this in the bath. When he is a few weeks old he may be placed on a blanket on the floor in a warm room and encouraged to kick and to be active.

Warmth

It is important to remember that a baby has a poorly developed heat-regulating centre and therefore needs to be kept warm in cold weather and cool if the weather turns very hot. A condition known as *neonatal cold injury* can occur in normal full-term babies born in the winter months, particularly between January and March. The baby is quiet and sleepy and difficult to feed but because the hands and feet and cheeks, although cold to the touch, are often pink it is not always realized that the baby is thoroughly cold. A new baby needs to be in a constant temperature of about 20°C (70°F) by day and night for the first few weeks after birth. A hot water bottle will warm the cot but must of course be removed before the baby is put in. It should be remembered that the room will be coldest in the small hours and even in summer the temperature drops quite sharply before dawn and many an adult pulls up an additional blanket at this time.

Clothing

Clothes for a baby should be light and warm and easy to put on and take off. Porous, non-irritating fabrics such as cotton and wool mixtures are best and the garments should not be restrictive. Garments in man-made fibres are easily laundered but are non-absorbent and may be too warm in summer or cause a heat rash on a sensitive skin. As they are changed every day ease of laundering is an important factor and many mothers favour a single all-in-one garment which can be undone to change the napkin whenever necessary. Alternatively a vest, gown and jacket may be worn. If mittens are needed care should be taken to see that there are no loose threads which can become wound round a finger and restrict the blood supply.

Welfare Clinic

A health visitor will be responsible for advising mothers about the care of a baby after the midwife has ceased to attend, or when the mother is discharged from hospital. All local authorities provide infant welfare clinics where the baby can be weighed, his progress assessed, and where he can be examined by the clinic doctor. Any problems relating to infant feeding and general child management may be discussed with the health visitor and opportunity also exists for health education to be given on a wide variety of topics. If medical treatment is found to be necessary, the child is referred to the general practitioner, hospital or appropriate special clinic, e.g. child guidance.

A special register known as the 'at risk' register is maintained by all local authority health departments. The register is a record of all children who are either born with some abnormality, or who develop some abnormality because of difficulties occurring in the antenatal, perinatal or postnatal periods. Such children are reviewed at frequent intervals by the clinic doctor until further check-ups are no longer felt to be necessary. The work of the clinic doctor lays emphasis on screening techniques and the early diagnosis of abnormality. Routine developmental assessments are made on all children at approximately three-monthly intervals during the first year, at 18 months and then yearly until the child is five. Toys and other equipment are used to test the development of particular skills and hearing and vision are also tested. An example of routine screening is the Guthrie test which is carried out in hospital or by the district midwife about the sixth day of life, for a condition called phenylketonuria which, if it remains undetected, gives rise to mental retardation, but which can be treated by diet if it is detected early enough. Another screening test, simply carried out, is one to exclude congenital dislocation of the hip (see Fig. 8).

In some areas where many mothers go out to work infant welfare clinics have been held in the evening. Because their mothers are usually in the lower income groups, children of immigrants make up a high proportion attending such clinics and they must be offered the same quality of preventive care as other members of society. Research has highlighted particular problems which occur frequently in immigrant

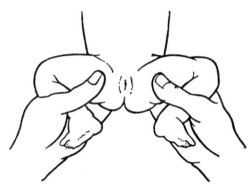

8. A test for congenital dislocation of the hip.

communities. Dietary difficulties are especially common. There exists a high rate of iron deficiency anaemia since iron-containing foods are not introduced into the diet early enough and there is a lack of understanding about food values. Similarly vitamin supplements are not added to the diet and deficiency diseases such as rickets frequently occur. Skin conditions, possibly related to climatic change, and a low resistance to upper respiratory tract infection are also seen. Failure to adapt to the cultural patterns of the host country may also give rise to psychiatric problems in immigrant mothers, depression being not uncommon, and to problems of child management. Many immigrant mothers may not understand the need for playing with and talking to their children since, in the country of their birth, child care may be undertaken by grandparents. Guidance and advice may be given about such problems at welfare clinics and an opportunity may also be created for the discussion of family planning where the mother may be too shy or isolated to know how to gain the information.

Immunization

Because the usual custom is to start an immunization programme during the first year the whole topic will be discussed here even though the programme will not be completed until the early teens.

To be effective immunizing practices must be extensively used throughout the community. The programme is less effective if started too early in infancy because the antibody-producing system will be too immature to make any adequate response. Contraindications to immunization include illness or any treatment which depresses antibody formation such as the administration of corticosteroids or irradiation, and two doses of any live vaccine should not be given within a month of each other.

Immunization against diphtheria, tetanus and pertussis (whooping cough) is usually combined as 'triple antigen'. Three separate injections are given about the ages of six months, seven to eight months and twelve months. At the same time oral poliomyelitis vaccine may be given by putting three drops on a spoon or a lump of sugar.

In the second year vaccination against smallpox is given if desirable. This is not given as a routine but in these days of rapid travel it is advisable for the children of parents who, because of their occupation or frequent international travel, may be at risk. Revaccination should be carried out every three years if there is risk of exposure to infection. At the end of the second year or early in the third, measles vaccination may be given to those children who have not had the disease. Only one dose is required.

A booster dose of triple antigen and of poliomyelitis should be given before the child starts school, at the age of four or five, or earlier if it is planned that the child should attend nursery school.

About the age of ten or eleven years primary school children are tested for their immunity to tuberculosis and if they have none they will be offered BCG (Bacille Calmette-Guerin) vaccine. This can of course be given in infancy if there is disease in the family. Girls may have vaccination against rubella (German measles) between the ages of eleven and thirteen years to prevent their contracting it during the first three months of pregnancy and the subsequent risk of congenital abnormality in the baby.

Children who have reached school leaving age may be given a further booster dose of triple antigen and poliomyelitis vaccine.

In some cases vaccination against influenza may be given to children with a chronic disorder which would become serious if they contracted influenza. Immunity is short-lasting and an annual booster dose is required.

Care in the Tropics

Immunization programmes in tropical countries follow a similar pattern to that described above but are started sooner. BCG vaccine is given in infancy and smallpox protection is given as a routine. An intermediate booster dose of triple antigen and poliomyelitis vaccine is usually given about the age of eighteen months in addition to those given before starting school and in many countries vaccination will also be given against typhoid, paratyphoid and yellow fevers and against cholera.

Maintenance of the health of babies and small children in the tropics is largely a question of keeping the child cool and preventing infection. A moses basket is better than a carry cot or pram and a soft rush mat can be placed over the mackintosh and below the bottom sheet to allow air to circulate more freely. One cotton cellular blanket is usually sufficient and in some countries a mosquito net will be required. A sponge bath is comforting in the evening as well as in the morning and cotton clothing will be the coolest, with long sleeves in the evenings where mosquitoes are a problem.

Breast feeding may be continued a little longer in the tropics if possible and older children will need frequent drinks of cool, boiled water.

Where there is a danger of malaria, mosquito-proofed windows and doors are essential and a net must be used at night. Regular spraying is helpful and a prophylactic drug such as pyrimethamine should be taken regularly. Areas in the immediate vicinity where mosquitoes or flies might breed should be cleared. Hookworm can be contracted by walking barefoot on infected ground so children should be taught to keep their shoes on, which also prevents injury due to thorns, etc. All drinking water should be boiled to prevent infestation with roundworm and children should only be allowed to bathe in swimming pools as ponds and streams may be infested with schistosomiasis.

Mental Health and Progress

The quality of parental care given from the beginning of a child's life is vitally important for his future mental health.

From birth, it is essential that the child should have a warm, continuous relationship with his mother or mother substitute, who can respond to his individual needs and provide continuity of care and experience. Research has shown that children deprived of this close mothering relationship during the first three years of life suffer intellectual retardation, speech impairment and show an inability to give or to receive affection. Such symptoms of emotional ill health lead to difficulties in making and sustaining satisfactory relationships in adult life and where there has been severe deprivation during childhood, signs of delinquency may develop.

Short periods of separation from the mother, such as occur when a small child is admitted to hospital, may also give rise to symptoms of anxiety and emotional upset in the child but lasting effects are not usually sustained if those looking after the child handle the situation wisely, by encouraging the mother to stay with her child and participate in his care.

It follows then that prolonged separation from the mother should be avoided if possible but if it is unavoidable, a mother substitute relationship and as homely an atmosphere as possible should be provided. The child who receives continuous loving care within a stable family unit eventually achieves the emotional security necessary for him to tolerate periods away from his mother, secure in the knowledge that she will return.

At first the new-born baby sleeps for the greater part of the 24 hours. He can suck, swallow, smell, taste and hear. He lies quietly when being cuddled by his mother, when being fed and when he feels warm and comfortable. He is able to remain alone for a short time only before a sense of loneliness may cause him to cry. Gradually he may become content to be alone for increasing periods if there is something he can see, such as his mother moving around the room or a coloured toy. While still very small he will be startled by loud noises and will like to be picked up firmly and supported well or he will feel insecure.

From as early as four weeks he will watch his mother's face intently as she feeds him and talks to him and by about six weeks he will begin to smile. Slowly he will begin to focus and move his eyes with some degree of coordination and by the age of three or four months he will begin to turn his head in the direction of sound. He now also recognizes his mother. By this time he is beginning to need more companionship and a longer playtime. He responds with pleasure to friendly handling, reacts to familiar situations and vocalizes when spoken to. By the age of six months his movements will be more controlled so that he can reach for a toy or can roll over when he is playing on the floor and sit up for a little while. His facial expression will be more responsive and by eight months he should be able to sit securely and will probably begin to pull himself up by a piece of furniture. The child's physical independence now gradually increases and he is constantly exploring and exploiting his environment but he remains closely dependent upon an adult's reassuring presence. The child who is living in a happy environment will make better progress at this stage than the child who is deprived of a stable home life. If the parents are interested and affectionate and are willing to play with the baby and encourage him to practise his new skills he will be happy and peaceful and will progress to the limits of his ability. No two children will progress at the same pace and comparisons should not be made.

Battered Babies and Cot Deaths

The so-called 'battered baby syndrome', or 'non-accidental injury to children', is a relatively new and largely unexplained phenomenon. Although the situation varies tremendously a typical picture is that of a well-cared-for child brought by anxious parents to the doctor or the hospital and found to have some of a wide variety of injuries ranging from simple bruising to fractures, sometimes including the skull (see Fig. 9).

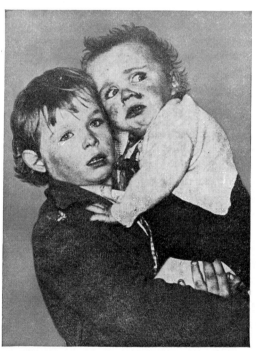

9. Battered children.

The explanation is given of a fall downstairs or a similar accident. The child is treated and returns home only to return later, or to be taken to a different doctor or hospital with further injuries. If the situation passes unnoticed, or is not investigated, the child may eventually die from his injuries. Investigation of such incidents is very difficult and the problem of how to deal with them remains. The important factor is the child, who must be removed from danger, if necessary by invoking the juvenile court.

'Battering' occurs in families of all social levels but frequently the parents are young and socially disabled. There may be a history of unemployment and criminal background and many are found to have a lower than average IQ. Other factors such as poor housing, overcrowding and marital instability may also be present. Frequently however it is discovered that the parents themselves were battered as children. In turn they become inadequate parents, seeking from their children the emotional comfort and gratification that they themselves were denied. The normal infant makes many demands which such parents are unable to meet and battering results, often as a form of punishment for persistent crying. Sometimes only one child in a family of several is affected.

Prevention depends on early detection of mental stress and the giving of adequate support and counselling where there is a known history of mental ill health.

Another cause of death which must be mentioned is the 'cot death' which occurs silently and unexpectedly, often during the night, to a child who was apparently perfectly well the previous day. The most common age for this to occur is about three months and there are probably more boys affected than girls. Because the event is more common in the winter months respiratory infection was thought to be a cause but research over twenty years has not shown any one single factor. Work is continuing to discover the cause and then to suggest some form of prevention. A death of this type naturally has a very traumatic effect on the parents who tend to blame themselves, or even each other.

3

The Toddler

Much of what has been said in Chapter 2 about the infant will also apply to the toddler although the routine of the day will begin to resemble more nearly that of the rest of the family.

Hygiene

It is customary for a toddler to have his daily bath in the evening before he goes to bed. If he has been actively enjoying and exploring his surroundings during the day he will be in need of it by the evening.

By the time he is one year old he will probably have about eight teeth and at this stage they should be very gently cleaned with a small, soft toothbrush and plain water. His diet should include crisp foods and those which require chewing; it is helpful to end each meal with a small piece of raw fruit such as apple, which has a cleansing action on the teeth, and finally a drink of water. When the teeth are cleaned it is important that they are brushed from the gums towards the biting surfaces and that a thorough rinsing should complete the process. Sometime between the ages of 2½ to 3 years a child should accompany his mother on one of her routine visits to the dentist to become familiar with the

routine and for the dentist to check for signs of early decay
or irregularity of the teeth. After this, visits should be arranged
at 4 to 6 monthly intervals.

Feeding

By the time the baby is about one year old he will be having
three meals a day with an extra drink given on waking
and when he goes to bed. He should be having a pint
of milk daily including that which is used in cooking.
He should not be allowed to 'nibble' between meals but
may if required have a drink or a piece of fresh fruit at
mid-morning.

He should be encouraged to feed himself whenever possible.
It is useful in many ways, particularly as the baby will eat
the amount he requires and not what the parent may assume
he requires. Proper preparation for self-feeding will make the
process more enjoyable and clearing up easier. A child who can
sit up should have his meals in a high chair which is placed
at the table with the rest of the family. In this way he learns
the social value of mealtimes. He must have a good-sized bib
or pinafore to protect his clothes and in the early stages it
may be necessary to cover the carpet with a washable mat.
This is preferable to letting the child eat his meals in the
kitchen before the rest of the family. Give him a teaspoon
and let him feed himself with whatever he can, though it
may be necessary to help him out rather than to let the food
get cold. It is easier for the child if the food is not too moist.
He has to be taught that the food is there to be eaten and not
to be played with. Toddlers are anxious to avoid 'missing
out' and this is particularly true of the extra carbohydrate
foods which many people enjoy. Ice-creams, crisps, biscuits,
sweets and sweet fruit drinks taken between meals will
satiate the small child's appetite and he may be unable to eat

the protein foods and vegetables he needs. Such luxury foods are best avoided or given as a treat immediately after meals and not as a between-meals snack.

Sleep and Exercise

At the age of one to two years the toddler is likely to sleep for 13 to 14 hours per day. Most of this will be at night but he will need to rest for one to two hours in the middle of the day and he will probably go to sleep then. As he gets older he may not sleep in the afternoon but should be encouraged to rest with a toy or a book. Always warn a child who is in the middle of a game that rest-time or bed-time are approaching and do not expect him to drop everything without warning. It is wise to shorten the afternoon rest gradually if the child is still having it by the age of $4\frac{1}{2}$ years so that he is used to being up all day by the time he starts school.

An active toddler will need plenty of opportunity to exercise his limbs; a play-pen may provide an environment where he can do this safely, though when he is supervised he can have more space to move about in. It is important that the child should be suitably clad for whatever activity he is likely to undertake so that his play, the only way in which he learns, is not spoiled by admonitions to mind his clothes. As much as possible of his exercise should take place in the fresh air and he should be out in the sun whenever possible though he will need protection from the direct rays.

Play

Play is one of the basic needs of all children and the provision of suitable play material, appropriate to the child's age, is important. Play has no single function. It aids in the overall development of body and mind and much can be learnt about a child's physical and emotional health from observing his play. The child distinguishes play from reality but uses objects and situations from the real world to create a world of his own. Play serves as an outlet for inner conflicts, e.g. throwing a doll onto the floor relieves feelings of jealousy about a new baby. Exciting or unpleasant events are repeated in play because repetition reduces the excitement which has been raised and also helps the child to come to terms with a disturbing situation by actively bringing it about rather than being a helpless spectator. This type of play is at its height between the ages of 18 months and 7 years; after this time, as thought processes mature, the child becomes better equipped to handle any difficult situations he may encounter. It is during this period that imaginary playmates are created and adult intrusions may be resented unless they became part of the make-believe framework. A great deal of play is imitative in nature and through this the child learns his social role. Little girls play at being 'mummy' and practise domestic chores, boys want to be involved in the more masculine activities associated with father. This type of play also promotes speech development since a child may be frequently heard to quote his parents when recreating a situation he has already experienced.

Play activity is also of intellectual value. It prevents boredom and helps the child to concentrate, to observe and to experiment. It enables the child to practise and develop new skills and teaches the use of hands and eye–hand coordination. Toys and games therefore which enable a child to practise new skills and to use his imagination are more likely to retain his interest over a long period.

Socially, play helps a child in his relationships with others, teaching him cooperation and the value of sharing his possessions. Outdoor play provides healthy exercise and opportunity for the practising of skills such as running, jumping and climbing.

The provision of play material should take into account the mental age of the child, his physical ability and his personal interests and aptitudes. When he can walk a large toy on wheels will give support and confidence and considerable pleasure. This may take the form of an animal such as a dog, or a barrow which can be loaded with a variety of objects and will be useful for games for some years. Balls and other round objects also encourage movement and activity.

By the age of 18 to 20 months the child will be increasingly mobile and his play area must be safe. He will be able to crawl up steps and stairs but not down and will be keen to climb on things, so windows must be guarded. Climbing encourages the use of limbs and helps to promote good balance but must be closely supervised.

It is ideal if there is a place in which he can play safely and in which he can do more or less what he likes. This helps to avoid the continual pleas for tidiness and the clearing up and putting away which is inevitable if the child must play in the family living room or kitchen.

Play is the only way to give a child practice in the activities which he will later require in earnest (see Fig. 10). It helps to develop both body and mind. Out of doors, water in a tub or large bowls will provide endless fascination and empty bottles, jugs, funnels, tubing, corks and other floating objects should also be provided. If there is room a sandpit with moulds, pails, spoons and spades will give many hours of enjoyment. Indoor play is slightly more restricted but small children love to 'help' with whatever household activity is taking place and will also like threading large beads, sorting buttons, playing with nuts and bolts and dressing up. Useful rubbish will provide occupation and scope for imagination and items such as cotton reels, empty cheese boxes, toilet roll cylinders, rubber bands, match boxes, string, clothes pegs, corrugated cardboard, pipe cleaners and coloured material can be saved up for production when a suitable time occurs. Until a child is old enough to appreciate the dangers he should not be given any article small enough to be swallowed or inserted into a body orifice.

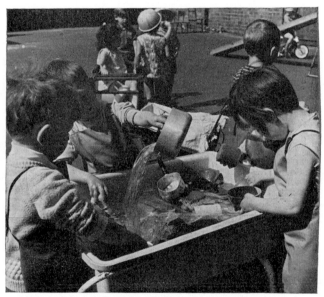

10. Playtime.

A great deal of play is imitative in nature. A child plays at being a bus conductor, a grocer or a dustman and in this way prepares himself to cope with a variety of situations as they occur. Many of these imaginative situations require the presence of an adult and time must be made during the day for playing with the small child.

Clothing

Clothing for the active toddler should be lightweight and not in any way restrictive. Since it will get heavy wear ease of laundering will be an important feature. A child should wear the minimum amount of clothing compatible with warmth— an extra pullover or cardigan can always be added when necessary. In cold weather long trousers, tights and anoraks are warm and easier to keep clean than overcoats. In warmer weather shorts or skirts worn with a shirt, and sandals with or without socks are sufficient.

Shoes must be chosen carefully and new ones bought whenever necessary so that foot growth is not cramped. Socks, too, can cramp toes if they are not big enough. It is early enough to buy the first shoes when the baby begins to walk and these should be flexible and roomy. He must wear them when walking on paths where there is grit and dirt, but at other times, indoors or on the beach he should be encouraged to go without them to encourage normal growth and development of the feet.

Tropics

In hot countries and in mid-summer in temperate countries cotton clothing is most suitable for a small child. In the late afternoon a cotton frock or blouse with long sleeves and long trousers may be necessary to guard against insect bites and as the temperature drops a light pullover may be needed. In glaring sun a hat is useful to protect the eyes.

As much extra fluid as required should be given in the form of cool boiled water with fruit juice, and added salt should be taken with meals. Fresh food which is to be eaten raw can be washed in Milton Solution 1–80 and rinsed in boiled water before serving.

To keep the skin fresh and free from 'heat rash' frequent cool showers or baths are refreshing, followed by a very light dusting with talcum powder.

Mental Health

Emotionally these early years can be very difficult. The small child has to learn how to use and control his increasing physical and mental power and he needs a great deal of help in this learning process. He requires quantities of love and his need for attention is so great that if he does not receive enough he is likely to behave badly in order to get it. It is better to be noticed for antisocial behaviour than not to be noticed at all. A parent who is nervous, quick-tempered and temperamental will not always get the best from a small child; the adult who has learned to control actions and emotions will find it easier to lead and guide a small child because so much is learned by example. The parent should endeavour to be consistent in the behaviour which is expected of the child and to try to avoid allowing him to do a thing one day and forbid it on another occasion. Behaviour which is clever and amusing in a tiny child on the first occasion will be less so if it is continued and may become quite objectionable in a four year old, yet if the child learns in the first instance that this behaviour is acceptable he cannot be expected to understand why it is not allowed later.

A child's love of approval is a useful weapon in the battle to encourage good behaviour and a sensitive child will respond quickly to a disapproving tone of voice at a very early age. On the whole it is better to teach the child by endeavouring to praise and approve good behaviour rather than punishing bad behaviour. The imposition of the adult's will should be reserved for those occasions on which the issue is really important and once a decision has been made it must be adhered to. No amount of wheedling or pleading by the child should alter the decision or the child will learn that if he keeps on long enough he will be allowed to have what he wants. Try to avoid offering a choice when there really is not one.

If he has to go to stay with Granny do not ask 'Would you like to stay with Granny?' but make it into a pleasurable statement of fact. Likewise a positive suggestion—to do something—is always better than a negative one—do not do something. A method of action which has been found by experience to bring success in childhood will remain into adult life and will colour dealings with other people. Thus, if in childhood it is found that throwing a tantrum is a successful means of getting one's own way it is likely that a similar type of behaviour will occur if one is thwarted in adult life. Similarly, if a child who craves attention finds that he gets it when he is ill he is likely to fall back on ill health as a way out of overwhelming difficulties in adult life. Illness in childhood should be treated as unlucky rather than as one long treat and a positive attitude should be adopted towards the full enjoyment of good health.

A small child will enjoy playing with his parents and should also be encouraged to play happily alone for increasing periods. Play with other children comes only gradually though he may get on well with an older child who gives him a lot of attention. Many only children need considerable help in learning the give and take which playing with other children requires and do not usually even begin to enjoy the company of other children until they are at least two years old.

Between one and two years of age a child is very dependent on its mother and enforced separations should be avoided as far as possible. The influence of the father is also very import-ant and will establish a basis for later relationships. Father represents strength and confidence to the child and provides love and companionship and emotional support for the mother, which are essential if she is to provide the contented atmosphere in which a child can thrive.

The average child begins to string words together between the ages of two to three years and will be helped by the mother talking to him, repeating common nouns and looking at pictures. Simple stories are usually enjoyed at this age. Once the child can talk he will begin to ask questions about the things which we take for granted but which to him are new and incomprehensible. If these questions are not answered his desire for knowledge will be frustrated and will eventually cease to exist. At the same time a very small child with a limited vocabulary may continue to ask 'Why?' simply as a means of continuing conversation when he is out of his depth and under these circumstances it may be wiser to help him out by suggesting an alternative occupation.

Accident Prevention

More accidents occur in the home than on the roads and the number of deaths is now over 8000 in every year. Small children and the elderly form by far the largest number of these tragedies. The toddler who has just found his feet and is curious about his surroundings is unaware of the danger which is close at hand (see Fig. 11).

Children's clothes should be made of non-flammable materials, particularly nightdresses and dresses. Fireguards should be placed round all fireplaces and should be firmly attached to the wall so that they cannot be pulled over. Free-standing electric fires and drip-feed heaters should not be used in homes where there are children and matches and candles for emergency use should be placed out of reach. In the kitchen care must be taken to turn the handles of pans

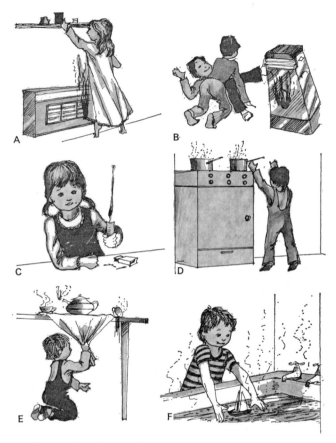

11. A, Unguarded fires are dangerous; B, Free standing heaters can be knocked over; C, Matches and candles are not toys; D, Projecting handles are a temptation; E, Tea and coffee can scald; F, A small child should not be alone in the bathroom.

away from the centre of the room. Special attachments may be bought to prevent the tipping over of saucepans on the stove and also to prevent gas taps being turned on inadvertently. Special care should be taken when serving out hot food or pouring tea when there is an active toddler in the room; a tablecloth which is hanging down and may be grasped for support is a potential danger. In the bathroom the cold water should be run into the bath before the hot and a small child must not be left alone in the bath.

Small children should not be given toys which have small detachable parts which they may inhale or swallow and great care must be taken not to leave plastic bags where a child can get at them (see Fig. 12).

Flexes trailing across the floor are dangerous and may cause a nasty fall. All electric sockets should be of the shuttered variety so that a child cannot poke anything into them. There are cases on record of accidents occurring with front-loading washing machines and with self-fastening refrigerators so care should be taken with these items.

All children like to climb and it may be necessary to fasten or bar upstairs windows so that it is impossible for a child to squeeze through.

Sharp knives and scissors are potential dangers and should be out of reach.

Of all cases of accidental poisoning admitted to hospital 80 per cent are children under five, most are aged between one and three. About 35 per cent of these cases originate in the kitchen from items such as disinfectants, bleaches and other household cleansers which are frequently stored in a low cupboard under the sink. They should be stored in a high cupboard and must never be transferred into empty milk or lemonade bottles. Poisoning with medicinal products is twice as common as with household products, salicylates being the most usual. Most drugs are stored in bedside or

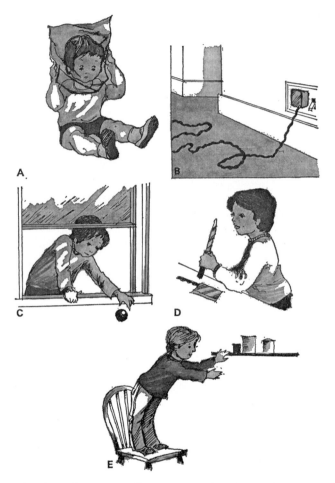

12. A, Plastic bags can suffocate; B, Trailing flex and unshuttered electric sockets are dangerous; C, Windows are a temptation; D, Sharp knives will cut; E, Medicines should be locked away.

dressing-table drawers or in bathroom cupboards which often cannot be locked. Where there are small children there should be a locking, or childproof, medicine cupboard. One reason for the frequency of accidental poisoning in children is the resemblance of many tablets to sweets and the sugar coating which surrounds them. It is normal for a small child to put things in his mouth and to imitate adults, so if parents are seen taking tablets the child may attempt to do the same. However, studies have shown that poisoning is most likely to occur in those families where there is environmental instability and parental disorder.

One other type of poisoning should also be mentioned here. Children living in old houses with flaking paint on woodwork and plaster or painted-over wallpaper and who also have 'pica'—the habit of eating unnatural substances—may develop lead poisoning. This can cause brain and kidney damage and may be fatal. Lead poisoning due to environmental factors is discussed in Chapter 14.

When so many families have a car the safety of the children during a drive is very important. A special safety seat should be provided, attached firmly to the rear seat and no journey should be made, however short, without the child being comfortably fastened in his seat.

The importance of a safe playing area has already been mentioned. Where a child is fortunate enough to have a garden to play in the gate should be capable of being securely fastened and all garden tools and pesticides must be safely put away.

All the precautions mentioned above are important and should be fulfilled if possible. They do not preclude, however, the need to teach the child, as soon as he is old enough, the correct use of the equipment so that he understands the dangers and the need to treat potentially dangerous items with respect.

Day Nurseries

Day nurseries are provided by Local Authorities to provide day care for young children who cannot remain at home because of their social circumstances. Mothers with young children under two years of age should be dissuaded from going out to work but nurseries should be available for those who must do so or who have very poor home conditions.

Ideally the nurseries should be close to the home or to the mother's work place and they should not take more than 40 to 50 children. There should be suitable premises and playgrounds staffed and equipped to ensure the physical well-being of the children and to prevent the spread of infection. The children are divided into small groups to resemble the family unit thus enabling them to gain some sense of security.

Private day nurseries must be registered with the Local Authority as must any person who looks after one or more children, to whom she is not related, in her own home.

One third of a pint of milk is provided free each day for each child attending a registered day nursery, play group or child minder.

Nursery Schools and Play Groups

Many parents send their children to nursery school or play group for a few hours once or twice a week, gradually extending it to every morning as the time comes for them to start school. In this way children become accustomed to being away from their mothers for a short while and to mixing with a number of other children. Most children enjoy the activities at nursery school and are then predisposed to going to school when the time comes.

4

The Schoolchild

Physical and Mental Health

At the age of five years the school life of the child begins and this creates a big change in the daily routine, but the child who has had an opportunity to attend nursery school or play group will adapt more easily to the large number of other children, the time spent without his mother and the restriction of his activity which school attendance will bring (see p. 48). He will settle down more easily too if, by the time he goes to school, he has learned to dress and undress himself, tie his shoe laces and attend to his own personal needs.

General Hygiene

A child at school should have a bath or all-over wash every day and this is probably most conveniently arranged before going to bed. By this age washing the hands before meals and after going to the lavatory should be established as a routine which the child can be depended on to carry out whether he is at school or at home. Teeth chould be cleaned morning and evening and after meals—if it is not possible to clean them after school dinner they should be brushed after breakfast and again when the child comes home in the afternoon. The hair should be brushed at least twice daily and combed when necessary. The frequency of hair washing will depend on the type of hair. A child at school must be taught to use only his own toilet articles and brush and comb and should be dissuaded from borrowing items such as hats, caps or gym shoes from other children.

Diet

There will be little change in the diet of the schoolchild except that his appetite may well increase with greater energy output. He needs a well-balanced diet with plenty of protein, which is necessary for growth. Each day's menu should also contain fresh fruit and fresh vegetables and one pint of milk each day including that which is used in cooking. A child at school should have a substantial breakfast before setting out and will probably like a snack and a drink when he arrives home in the afternoon. The last meal of the day should not be too heavy and should not be served too near bedtime. No meals should be eaten in a hurry so the child should be up in good time to eat breakfast and if he comes home to lunch it should be ready when he comes in. Schoolchildren are particularly likely to eat too many carbohydrate foods and obesity is a common form of malnutrition among children in this country. The amount of sweets, crisps and other carbohydrate foods they eat should be restricted and the hungry child may be encouraged to have a drink of milk or some fresh fruit as an alternative.

Rest and Recreation

Children starting school are likely to be tired at the end of the day and require a good night's rest. In addition to the length of the day, during which they are learning and concentrating, there is the added strain of mixing with many other children. Some children require a period of rest and quiet as soon as they come home and this can be conveniently combined with a drink and a snack in many cases. Children vary considerably in the amount of sleep they require and the best guide is their readiness to get up in the morning. The child who has to be woken every morning from a deep sleep is not having long enough and should go to bed earlier. Between the ages of 5 and 7 years 11 to 12 hours is usually needed and up to the age of 11 many children require 10 to 11 hours' sleep.

Between school and bedtime the child should be encouraged to follow his own interests and part of this time should be spent in the fresh air if the weather is suitable. Many children like to join one of the many youth organizations which may give them an opportunity to meet children other than those they meet at school. If there is homework this should be completed early in the evening so that it is finished and there is time for a change of occupation before bed. A separate place should be provided if this is possible so that both the child and the family can follow their own pursuits without interruption.

There are strict regulations regarding the employment of children, but these vary from one area to another. Generally they must not take a job at all under the age of thirteen. In some areas over this age they may work for one hour only before school, in other areas any work may only be done after school hours. Work may not begin before 6 am or continue after 8 pm and a child may not work for more than two hours on Sunday or on any school day.

Clothing

Perhaps the single most important factor in the selection of clothes for schoolchildren is that they should be easily washed.

Most children enjoy wearing school uniform but if this is not the custom it is advisable to have suitable clothes kept for school wear and something different to wear at weekends. Clothes should be comfortable and allow freedom of movement and be of a suitable weight for the season.

Mental Health

The 'opening up' of a child's life which accompanies going to school provides a great deal of new stimulus, excitement and some anxiety. The child is venturing out into a less sheltered world and at this time he needs parents who will help him towards independence, but who will also continue to provide a warm, secure home background. Initially, although still basically self-centred, the child will work and play with others in small groups, and he begins to learn, through such social interaction, the value of sharing achievements, satisfactions and disappointments. Despite his growing independence the child still needs adult guidance and during the first years at school teachers act as parent substitutes, controlling the child's activity and giving appropriate encouragement. Children in the five to seven age group are full of energy and eager to learn and it is important to see that they do not become overtired.

Between the ages of eight and eleven, the child becomes increasingly independent of adults, group activity assumes greater importance and the child derives companionship and emotional satisfaction from contact with his friends.

The child is also showing considerable intellectual progress. He can now clearly distinguish fact from fantasy and the ability to think logically is developing. Skill in reading is gradually acquired and parents should encourage this. The child at this time is very anxious to learn and both school and home should provide stimulating, rewarding activity. He needs also firm, decisive and consistent guidance from parents and teachers which leaves him free to explore his environment and make decisions for himself.

All children react differently to the experiences encountered when they first enter school life. Many children want to share their new experiences and cannot get the words out quickly enough to tell all that they have been doing. Other children seem almost overwhelmed by school happenings and are unable to share them with their parents. It is important not to drag information unwillingly from such a child but to give him the love and support he needs and to show interest in whatever information he does proffer. The mother should always be at home when the child leaves for school and when he returns.

During the first years at school a child needs to become an accepted member of a group and to learn the value of co-operative living with his family, friends and classmates. The comfort and support of parents is vital since it prepares the child to withstand the stress of puberty. It is necessary too that parents recognize the child's potential and do not over-estimate his capacity for academic achievement. Pushing the child beyond his capabilities, 'babying' him or displaying too little parental authority may cause failure in learning and in the child's ability to adapt to his social environment.

School Health Services

Concern about the health of young people began when young men, recruited to serve in the Boer War, were medically examined; over 50 per cent of them had to be rejected because they were suffering from serious medical defects of one sort or another. Various measures were adopted to improve the

health of the young and among them was the gradual formation of the school health service.

The aims of the service are to make sure that every child is
as fit as possible and so gain the greatest benefit from his
education. Particular attention is paid to the early diagnosis
of any disability in order that treatment can be started before
the condition becomes irremediable. In addition to the
preventive aspects of the service there is also a positive effort
to improve health. The service is also responsible for the
diagnosis and treatment of handicapped children.

An important part of the service is the maintenance of
accurate records about each child. The record from the Infant
Welfare Clinic is passed on to the school health service when
the child begins school and in this way an uninterrupted
medical history is available. The records from the general
practitioner may also be made available if necessary.

Medical examinations are carried out at schools maintained
by the Local Education Authorities. The first examination is
usually shortly after the child enters the infant school, though
some authorities are trying out a system whereby each child
is seen one year before starting school to enable any defect to
be diagnosed and treated before the child commences school.
A dental examination at this time enables preventive dental
treatment to be started early if necessary. About 14 per cent
of children are found to have some medical defect when they
start school. Parents are always invited to attend the medical
examination and a careful medical history is taken which,
together with the child health centre records and a note of
the health of the family, provides the doctor with a complete
story of the child's progress during the preschool years. A
full medical examination is then carried out and if any treatment is required it is usually obtainable at the local hospital,
after the general practitioner has been informed. Eyesight

and hearing are both tested and if they are found to be defective the child is referred to the appropriate department for further investigation and treatment. At the conclusion of the examination a record is made and the doctor indicates when he would like to see the child again.

In some areas all children are seen routinely on entering school, at transfer to senior school and on leaving school. In other areas a *selective medical examination* system is in operation in which all children are examined thoroughly on entry and parents are asked to fill in a questionnaire relating to the child's health when he is eight and when he is twelve years old. A further medical examination is carried out if the answers to the questionnaire reveal that this is necessary, if the parent, teacher or school nurse request that the child is seen or if there is a history of repeated absence from school. A child who has a chronic disability would be seen by the doctor at his annual visit to the school and a previously healthy child who develops a severe illness would also be seen annually or as necessary. Children 'at risk' are also seen as necessary, usually more often than the normal child.

School dental inspections are carried out annually or every six months and if treatment is required this may be performed at the school clinic or the child may be referred to his own dentist. In rural areas a mobile clinic is used to prevent too much time being lost away from school. Orthodontic treatment is also carried out for children who require it and must be started early enough so that permanent teeth may develop correctly.

In some areas the school nurse runs a *minor injuries clinic* at which schoolchildren can be treated, while in others a child must attend its own general practitioner or the local hospital.

Regular inspections of the children are undertaken by the school nurse for *cleanliness* or signs of infestation (see Chapter 5). About 2 per cent of schoolchildren are found to be infested with head or body lice and in these cases cleansing is undertaken. At the same time the family must be visited to ensure that other members of the family are treated if necessary. If this is not done the child will become reinfested. Infestation occurring repeatedly in the same family must be investigated and if it is found to be due to neglect the parents may be liable to a fine.

A child who has behavioural difficulties may be referred for help to a *child guidance clinic* where a team of psychiatrists, educational psychologists and psychiatric social workers will try to establish the cause of such difficulty and to assist the child to overcome it. A child may be referred to such a clinic by the school medical officer, the family doctor or by the head teacher of his school.

The social development of the schoolchild may be looked after by an *education welfare officer* or *social worker*. Many problems to do with progress at school, clothing and uniform grants, maintenance allowances and help with the cost of school meals or transport are within the sphere of this officer and he is particularly concerned with unsatisfactory attendance records of individual children. Many authorities have now introduced an integrated service which links together child guidance, school psychological, remedial teaching and education welfare personnel into a *social education team* whose responsibility is to detect and correct any factor which comes between, or interferes with the child and his educaton.

The responsibilities of the school medical team do not end with the medical examination of children. They are also responsible for the *investigation of outbreaks of infectious disease* and prevention of spread if possible. If a case of tuberculosis occurs in a school all contacts among both staff and children must be examined and X-rayed or tuberculin tested as necessary. The *immunization* of those children who need it and the administration of booster doses where necessary is carried out by the school medical team and they are responsible also for the general supervision of *health education*. This should fit naturally into the school curriculum and will include such topics as dental hygiene, smoking and health, immunization, sex education and the encouragement of active participation in sport. A further duty of the medical team is periodic inspection of the school premises for standards of hygiene, paying particular attention to the state of the buildings, the lavatory and washing facilities and the cleanliness of the kitchens.

School Meals and Milk

Midday meals are provided for children attending local authority schools. These are subsidized and cost very little; financial help is also available in cases of hardship. Free milk is provided for children in nursery and infant schools up to the end of the summer term following their seventh birthday and for children attending special schools. Certain children may have it if the school medical officer certifies that it is necessary and for other children it is available at an economical price.

Handicapped Children

The detection and care of the handicapped child is an important part of the health care of the nation. The type and extent of the handicap varies greatly from one child to another but there are certain principles of care which apply to all handicapped children. It is important that the degree of handicap is *diagnosed as early as possible*. This is particularly important in cases such as deafness which should be discovered within the first year of life. Special *education should be started early*—as soon as it is diagnosed in cases of deafness, at about the age of two for the blind and before the age of five for many others. The school leaving age for handicapped children is sixteen years. The aim should be to make each child as independent and able to live as normal a life as is possible; success in adult life often depends on the degree of independence attained in childhood. It is a mistake to treat the handicapped differently and the best solution to any problem will always be the one which is as near normal as possible. Handicapped children may be educated in a normal school with healthy children or in a special class. Alternatively they may attend a special school as a day or boarding pupil.

Blindness

Blind children are those who have no useful sight. Many start their education at the age of two in nursery schools run by the Royal National Institute for the Blind. Most older children attend special residential schools for the blind, though some large cities have day schools. Partially sighted children are often taught in special day schools or in special classes in ordinary schools where classes are small and special equipment is available.

Deafness

Deaf children must start their education and training as soon as diagnosed and most older children attend residential schools where specialized tuition may enable them to learn to talk. Partially hearing children are helped with hearing aids and may attend special small classes in ordinary primary and secondary schools.

Delicacy

Delicate children who are particularly liable to become ill may attend special schools as day pupils or they may go to a residential school. This is particularly likely when an assessment of the child's condition is to be made, after which and following the completion of any special treatment, the child may be able to return home and attend a day school. Unsatisfactory home conditions may necessitate the child's staying on at a residential school; where education has been interrupted frequently and the child has become backward, an over-protective attitude on the part of the parents will only further handicap the child.

Educational Subnormality

Children who are educationally subnormal are educated at special schools or in special classes at normal schools. There is a very fine line dividing the child of low average intelligence from the educationally subnormal child; concentration, motivation and training can affect performance markedly. Repeated testing and careful obervation of the child in a special class or school by an experienced teacher will be necessary before a decision can be made about the correct type of education for any particular child. It may be better for a child to be educated in a special school to the upper limit of his own ability than to be continually at the bottom of his class and left behind his schoolfellows. Behaviour problems and juvenile delinquency are more common among children of lower intelligence and the school health service and the educational welfare service are continually working to reduce this problem.

Older children who are mentally subnormal attend junior training centres on a daily basis. They are taken by bus from a collecting point near their homes or in some cases, particularly in rural areas, they may be resident from Monday to Friday, returning home at weekends. Training centres concentrate on social training and the fostering of independence.

Habit training, table manners, care of clothes and personal hygiene all form an important part of the regime and group activities such as acting, games and playing in a percussion band.

Maladjustment

Maladjusted children are those who may become retarded educationally in spite of good or average intelligence, because of their behavioural difficulties. The causes of maladjustment may be many and include such factors as emotional instability, psychological disorders, unstable home conditions and marital difficulties between the parents, or a combination of two or more of these factors. These children may be educated in residential schools but if it is at all possible they benefit from the contact with normal children which they would get by attending a normal school. They will be fully investigated and treated by the staff of the Child Guidance Clinic and the treatment and support may continue over many years. Failure with a maladjusted child may have serious consequences as he may drift into criminal behaviour.

Physical Handicap

Physically handicapped children are educated in residential special schools or in special day schools if there is one close enough. Independence is encouraged and if possible they should attend an ordinary school as soon as they are able.

Epilepsy

Epiletic children can be educated normally provided that the child is emotionally stable and the fits do not occur too often. The teaching staff must be sympathetic and have good liaison with the school doctor. There are special schools for those children who are not acceptable at an ordinary school and after assessment and treatment in such a school some children may be able to return to an ordinary school.

Speech Defects

Children who have a speech defect should be educated at an ordinary school whenever possible. Speech therapy should be given at an early age and teachers must appreciate that a child who cannot make himself understood will become frustrated which will increase his speech defect and cause emotional difficulties. There are some conditions associated with an inability to understand words which may make normal education impossible and these children require special educative facilities.

Autism

The autistic child also requires special educational facilities and is frequently found in a school for subnormal children though 15 to 20 per cent of autistic children score normally in intelligence tests which do not involve language. These children also have difficulty in understanding non-verbal communication such as a smile, an expression of impatience or a warning frown.

Gifted Children

In recent years it has become increasingly realized that children who have a particular gift or ability and those with an intelligence which is considerably above average also require special education suited to their ability. There are schools for children with one special talent such as music, dancing, acting or other gifts but the child with a general ability usually has to manage with teaching designed for children older than himself. This is being overcome in some areas by the formation of group sessions in which intelligent children from a number of schools are able to get together and enjoy each other's stimulus and company.

Voluntary Societies

In addition to the health, social and educational services provided by the local authorities there are many voluntary organizations which provide aid and advice for handicapped children and their families. The parents of a child with a specific handicap should be advised to get in touch with the society dealing with that condition so that they gain support from contact with the society and with other families who have a similar problem. One society is the Invalid Children's Aid Association which helps any sick or crippled child and advises the family about available welfare services. Moral support is given wherever it is needed and in some cases financial help may be made available. Both parents and children benefit from meeting others like themselves and the brothers and sisters of handicapped children are not forgotten. The Association runs two schools for children who suffer from asthma and two for children with speech and language difficulties, There is also a 'word blind' centre for dyslexic children. The school fees for children needing this type of special education would be paid for by the Local Authority in the area where the child lives.

5

Health Education I

The health education of children (as mentioned in Chapter 4) should fit naturally into the school curriculum so that they learn that there is much that can be done by the individual towards the maintenance of his own health. They must be taught also about the consequences of neglect.

Personal Hygiene

The Skin

The skin has many functions which make it more than just the outer covering of the body but it is unable to carry out these functions effectively if it is not kept clean. After a normal day, the skin has accumulated debris in the form of dried sebum from the sebaceous glands, salts from evaporated sweat, dust, bacteria and scales of dead cells. On hot days or following exercise when sweating has been excessive and in dusty areas, there is a greater accumulation of debris. The skin should be washed all over every day, using hot water and soap and then dried thoroughly. This removes the substances from the skin which, if left there to be acted on by bacteria, cause the characteristic body odour which is so unpleasant for other people. A shower is the most economical and effective way of washing all over; a warm bath has the added value of being relaxing and is therefore soothing before going to bed; many people have neither of these facilities and manage effectively with a bowl of hot water.

Most women and many men require a good deodorant/ antiperspirant which is applied to the axillae where, because two skin surfaces are in close proximity, the warm moist area makes an ideal breeding ground for bacteria. There are many effective and inexpensive products on the market and the best one for any individual is a matter of personal choice, but none can be effective on unwashed skin. Girls must be taught to cleanse the perineal area when they have been to the lavatory, starting from the pubic area and working towards the anal area. Each piece of toilet paper should be used once only. This helps to reduce the likelihood of infecting the urinary tract with organisms from the anal area such as *Escherichia coli*.

Neglect of personal hygiene increases the likelihood of infestation with parasites of various types.

The *body louse* (*Pediculus corporis* see Fig. 13A) is a light grey insect that lives in clothing, particularly in seams or folds. It bites the body and sucks the blood causing intense irritation. The scratching which follows the bite causes secondary infection which may lead to septic dermatitis. Lice may also carry the organisms which cause diseases such as typhus, relapsing fever and trench fever. The female lays eggs (nits) which are cemented to hairs or to clothing and are themselves hatched and mature within 4 weeks. Infestation is less likely to occur if baths are taken regularly and clothing and bed-clothes are washed regularly. If it does occur, cleansing is carried out by giving a thorough bath and dusting the body with 10 per cent DDT powder before putting on clean clothes. The rest of the family should also be investigated and treated if necessary to prevent reinfestation. Clothing is treated with moist heat (100°C for 1 hour) and underclothes should be ironed with a hot iron to kill any nits which may be in the seams.

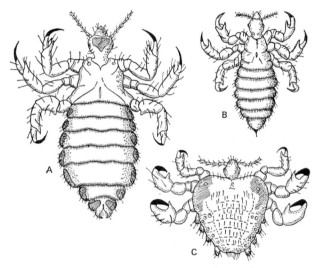

13. A, Body louse; B, Head louse; C, Pubic louse (showing relative sizes).

The *pubic louse* (*Pediculus pubis* see Fig. 13C) is also called the crab louse because it is said to resemble a crab. This lives in the pubic hair or other short hair on the body and may transmit the same diseases as the body louse. The treatment is as for body lice though, in addition, the infested hair may be shaved.

Fleas (*Pulex irritans* see Fig. 14) are wingless insects that live on the blood they suck after biting the host. Minute specks

of brown dried blood on sheets, pyjamas or underwear may
be present and will help to establish which parasite is causing
infestation. Fleas have strong back legs which enable them to

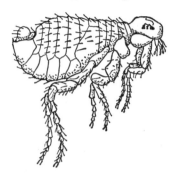

14. Flea.

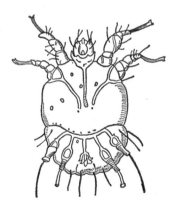

15. Scabies mite.

jump considerable distances. The common flea does not carry
disease but the bite is very irritating and causes scratching
and lack of sleep and the bites may become infected. Eggs are
laid in bedding, dust or rubbish and cracks in floors and the

partially developed flea may lie dormant for long periods
before completing its life cycle. Cleanliness of clothes and
body does a great deal to prevent infestation but if it does
occur accidentally, a thorough bath should be taken and DDT
applied to the clothes. An infested room or building should
be cleared of old bedding, carpets and clothing and dust and
dirt. It should then be thoroughly scrubbed and aired and

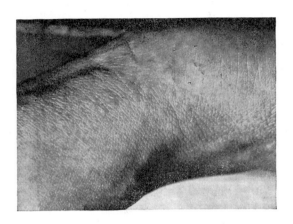

16. Scabies.

DDT powder can be blown into cracks round walls and
floors, and into furniture. The rat flea (*Xenopsylla cheopsis*)
may be responsible for transferring plague organisms from
rats to man.

The female *scabies mite* (*Sarcoptes scabei*) burrows into the
skin and lays eggs at the end of the burrow, causing intense
irritation which is worse at night. The male remains on the
surface of the skin. The scratching usually causes secondary
infection and an infected impetigo follows. The mite (see Fig.
15) is spread by close contact; it is common to find more than
one person in a household infested at the same time. The

treatment of scabies is to give a thorough bath and then to apply benzyl benzoate solution 25 per cent over the whole body from the neck down. When it is dry, a second application is made. Other members of the family must be treated at the same time.

The Hair

The importance of brushing the hair thoroughly twice daily and washing it as often as necessary has already been mentioned. The brush and comb should be washed thoroughly whenever the hair is washed and each individual should always use his own.

The *head louse* (*Pediculus capitis* see Fig. 13B) is more likely to be found on the heads of those whose hair is not kept clean, although accidental infestation can also occur. The insect resembles the body louse but is smaller and the eggs (nits) are stuck on to the hair close to the scalp with a cement-like substance. Common sites to find them are at the nape of the neck and behind the ears. Scratching, due to the intense irritation, may cause the bites to become infected and this in turn may cause swelling of the glands at the back of the neck and infected impetigo. Treatment is to apply a substance containing 0·5 per cent malathion to the scalp and allowed to dry *without* the use of heat; about 24 hours later the hair may be washed and then combed with a fine toothed comb. A weak solution of acetic acid may be required to remove the nits; treatment must be continued until all nits have been dealt with or reinfestation will occur.

Ringworm (*Tinea*) is a fungal parasite that attacks hair follicles and destroys the hairs which break off leaving balding, scaly patches which are usually circular or ring-shaped. The condition is very contagious and those affected should remain apart until the condition has cleared. Treatment involves the removal of diseased hairs, treating the diseased patches and the administration of oral drugs, such as griseofulvin. All personal items such as brushes and combs should be destroyed as it is almost impossible to ensure that they are free of spores.

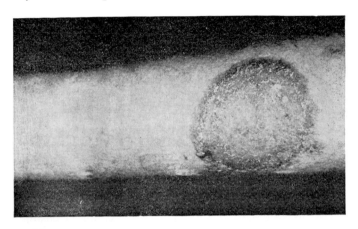

17. Ringworm.

The Feet

The feet must be kept scrupulously clean by frequent washing and careful drying between the toes. Feet perspire a great deal and a clean pair of socks or stockings should be worn every day. Shoes should be aired well after wearing and ideally there should be two pairs in use to be worn on alternate days and allowed 24 hours to air before they are worn again. Toenails should be kept trimmed and should be cut straight across as this helps to reduce the risk of ingrowing toe nails which can be very painful (see Fig. 18).

A troublesome condition known as *athlete's foot* (*Tinea interdigitalis*) is caused by a fungal infection between the toes and the infection may be spread by the use of communal bath mats and towels, and in changing rooms and swimming pools. Drying thoroughly between the toes helps to prevent the infection and children should be taught to step out of

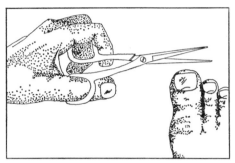

18. The correct method of cutting toenails—straight across.

the bath straight into their own slippers or shoes, if they are in the position of having to use communal changing facilities.

The Hands

Hands must be kept scrupulously clean to avoid the risk of infection. Mention has already been made of the importance of washing the hands before meals and after going to the lavatory. They must also be dried carefully to reduce the risk of roughness and cracking of the skin which provides an opening through which infection may enter. The use of a good hand or barrier cream will help to keep the skin in condition and is particularly useful in the winter months when 'chapping' is more likely. The fingernails must be kept short and clean and should be filed to the shape of the finger ends. Very shortly after it has been applied, nail varnish cracks and can harbour pathogenic organisms so it should not be worn by those whose jobs entail handling of food or contact with ill people.

The Teeth

Teeth should be cleaned night and morning and after meals. Brushing should be carried out away from the gums towards the biting surface which helps to sweep away food debris

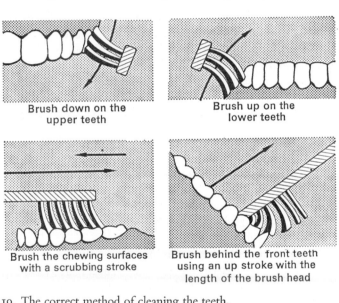

Brush down on the
upper teeth

Brush up on the
lower teeth

Brush the chewing surfaces
with a scrubbing stroke

Brush behind the front teeth
using an up stroke with the
length of the brush head

19. The correct method of cleaning the teeth.

from between the teeth and also stimulates the gums (see Fig. 19). Visits to the dentist for a check-up should be arranged at a minimum of six-monthly intervals. Neglect of the teeth can lead to infection in the mouth and in other parts of the body as well as being unpleasant for other people if halitosis develops. Fluorine is valuable in the prevention of tooth decay and in some areas it is added to the water supply for this reason. Where this has been done, there has been a substantial reduction in the amount of dental caries (see Chapter 11).

Food and Fluids

Good health is dependent on satisfactory nutrition. Substances which can serve as food for the body are those which it can use as fuel for providing warmth and energy and those which provide building material for the repair and growth of tissues. All animals require these building materials for the repair of body tissues which are constantly active and are being worn out by this activity; in addition, children require extra building material to build up the new tissues needed for growth.

Personal Requirements

There are six essential foodstuffs which must be constantly supplied to the body through the food which is eaten (see Fig. 20).

Proteins are essential for building up cell protoplasm and are therefore necessary for growth and repair. They are found in both animal and plant matter but the animal proteins are most valuable to the human body as building material, since they are similar to human protein in composition. The sources of protein are:

(1) Animal protein—meat, fish, eggs, cheese and milk
(2) Plant protein—wheat, rye, peas and beans.

Unfortunately, animal proteins are expensive so that people

Essential Food Requirements

An estimated 2000 calories a day are needed to maintain basic body functions and replace heat loss. The normal diet contains about 3000 calories a day, but a manual worker may need as much as 4000–5000 calories.

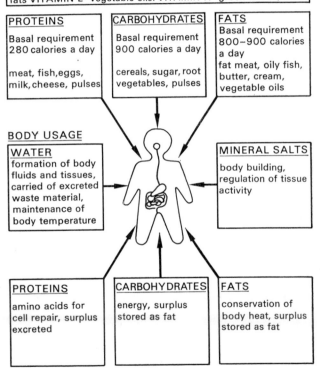

VITAMINS CONTAINED IN A BALANCED DIET
VITAMIN A—animal fats, green vegetables. VITAMIN B—cereals, pulse foods, yeast. VITAMIN C—fresh fruit. Vitamin D—animal fats VITAMIN E—vegetable oils. VITAMIN K—green leaves, liver.

PROTEINS	CARBOHYDRATES	FATS
Basal requirement 280 calories a day	Basal requirement 900 calories a day	Basal requirement 800–900 calories a day
meat, fish, eggs, milk, cheese, pulses	cereals, sugar, root vegetables, pulses	fat meat, oily fish, butter, cream, vegetable oils

BODY USAGE

WATER	MINERAL SALTS
formation of body fluids and tissues, carried of excreted waste material, maintenance of body temperature	body building, regulation of tissue activity

PROTEINS	CARBOHYDRATES	FATS
amino acids for cell repair, surplus excreted	energy, surplus stored as fat	conservation of body heat, surplus stored as fat

VITAMINS Vitamin A—growth, resistance to infection. Vitamin B— nutrition of nerve cells, red corpuscles. Vitamin C—wound healing. Vitamin D—regulates calcium absorption. Vitamin K— formation of prothrombin.

20. Daily basic food requirements for health.

on restricted incomes, such as pensioners, find it difficult to buy sufficient for their needs. It is worth remembering that the cheaper cuts of meat and fish have just as good a food value as the more expensive, though they may need more preparation. Some of both animal and plant proteins should be taken every day; egg, fish or meat could be taken at breakfast time and another animal protein at each of the other main meals.

Carbohydrates are the chief sources of body fuel and include starch and sugar. The sources of starch are cereals, root vegetables such as potatoes and parsnips and peas, beans and lentils. Sugar comes from sugar cane and sugar beet, all sweet vegetables, fruit and honey. If more carbohydrate is eaten than is required for warmth and energy it is converted into body fat and stored in the fat depots.

Fat also serves as body fuel and is obtained in the form of animal fat from fat meat and oily fish and from dairy products such as butter, milk and cream. It can also be obtained from vegetable oils such as are used to make margarine. Animal fats are more useful as food because they contain vitamins A and D, although all margarine manufactured today is treated to ensure adequate supplies of these vitamins.

Water forms two-thirds of the body and is present in most of the food we eat. In addition to that contained in food the body needs two to three litres of water every day to help in the formation of body fluids and tissues, to act as a carrier for the excreted waste material from metabolism, to cool the body by the evaporation of sweat and to prevent constipation.

Mineral salts are required for body building and are also regulators of tissue activity. Sodium, potassium and phosphorus and other trace elements are present in adequate amounts in a normal diet. Calcium, iron and iodine are the only minerals likely to be insufficient. Calcium is found mainly in milk and cheese and an adequate intake of vitamin D is needed for its utilization. Iron is obtained from green vegetables, red meat and egg yolk and is necessary to prevent certain types of anaemia. Iodine is present in seafood and is required for the normal functioning of the thyroid gland.

Vitamins are also essential to normal health and without them deficiency diseases may occur. Vitamins A, D, E and K are fat-soluble vitamins and are found in fat-containing foods. Vitamin C and the B group are water-soluble. *Vitamin A* is present in animal fats and, in a slightly different form, in green and yellow vegetables and fruit. It is necessary for normal growth in children and for normal vision. It also helps the body to resist infection. *Vitamin B* is really a group of vitamins which all come from a similar group of foods. They are present in 'wholemeal' cereals and in yeast and yeast extracts. To a lesser extent they are also found in vegetables, fruit, milk, eggs and meat. They contribute to general growth and the health of nerve tissue and a gross deficiency of the B vitamins is not common in this country. *Vitamin C* is present in fresh fruit and vegetables though it is largely destroyed by cooking and by storing for long periods, so fresh fruit or salad should be included in the daily diet. There is so little vitamin C present in milk that a baby being fed on cow's milk should be given supplementary vitamin C. It is necessary in the prevention of infection. *Vitamin D* is present in animal fats and is also manufactured in the skin when it is exposed to sunlight. It is important for the normal development of bones and teeth. *Vitamin E* is present in vegetable oils but little is known of its importance in human beings. *Vitamin K* can be obtained from green vegetables and from liver and is synthesized in the intestines. It is necessary for the manufacture of prothrombin and is therefore necessary for the normal clotting of blood.

Roughage is indigestible and remains in the bowel, stimulating peristalsis and thus preventing constipation. It forms the fibrous part of vegetables and fruit and is present in wholemeal flour.

The **value of food** is rekoned by the amount of heat which it yields on combustion. The heat is measured in *kilocalories*: 1 k/c is the amount of heat required to raise the temperature of 1 kilogram of water through 1°C.

1 gram of protein gives 4 kilocalories; 1 gram of carbohydrate gives 4 kilocalories; and 1 gram of fat gives 9 kilocalories.

An average diet should provide 2500 to 3000 k/calories per day, of which about 280 k/c should be provided by protein (70 g) and about 900 k/c by fat (100 g). The remainder would be provided by carbohydrate (300 to 400 g). More protein is required by children, by expectant mothers and by anybody leading a very active life such as athletes, or a man working at a heavy manual job. A varied diet which includes meat, fish, dairy products, vegetables and fresh fruit will provide vitamins and adequate nourishment to maintain health. In developing and over-populated countries, lack of animal protein and fat is responsible for a low standard of health. In western countries obesity is the most common form of malnutrition and it is usually due to excessive carbohydrate intake, frequently in the form of sweets, crisps, cakes and pastry. Obesity in children is an increasing problem and has been mentioned already in connection with baby feeding. Obesity is linked with a high incidence of coronary thrombosis, diabetes and osteoarthritis and tends to aggravate, and hinder recovery from, many other pathological conditions.

Many factors affect the dietary intake needed by an individual. Children require more because they are growing, in addition to being very active. A man requires more than a woman and a person of heavier build requires more than a slight person, unless the extra weight is due to fat. A smaller intake will be adequate in hot climates and in hot weather.

Care of Food in the Home

A refrigerator is the most satisfactory place to store perishable foods, but if one is not available, food must be kept cool and covered in a well-ventilated larder. Failing this, items such as milk and butter can be placed in a container standing in a bowl of water and surrounded by a cover of unglazed pottery, foam or muslin, which is also in contact with the water (see Fig. 21). The water will soak up through the porous cover

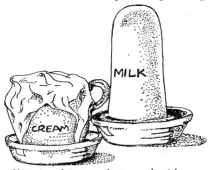

21. Methods of keeping dairy products cool without a refrigerator.

and the food will be kept cool by evaporation. Insulated containers such as those made of expanded polystyrene are useful for storing small amounts of food.

Food that has been deep frozen must be completely thawed before use and then thoroughly cooked to ensure that any *Salmonella* organisms, if present, are destroyed.

Milk should be taken indoors as soon as possible and the bottle must be wiped with a damp cloth before being placed in the refrigerator. All shelves and cupboards where food is stored must be cleaned frequently. Flies are a particular hazard if food is left uncovered and a kitchen should be kept as free of flies as possible.

The hands must be washed immediately before preparing food and again if it is necessary to answer the door, change the baby or blow the nose in the middle of cooking. Food which is to be reheated must be heated quickly and eaten immediately and hot food which is to be stored must be cooled quickly and then kept cold. Food which is kept warm is most likely

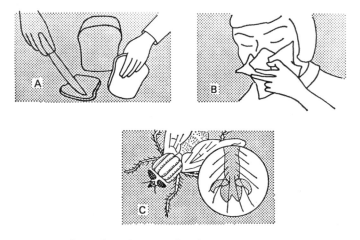

22. Ways of spreading disease A, hands—in contact with septic spots, boils and other infections deposit microorganisms on food; B, Coughs and sneezes—staphylococcal infections of nose and throat are readily spread by means of droplets; C, Flies—microorganisms adhere to the minute hairs of a fly's foot (inset) from which they can be transferred to food.

to cause food poisoning because the causative organisms are given the temperature, moisture and time they need to multiply to dangerous proportions. All fruit, vegetables, salad, fish and meat should be washed before being prepared. Kitchen surfaces should be covered with an easily cleansed and impermeable material such as adhesive plastic; this is readily available in the shops in a variety of attractive colours and patterns. Wooden surfaces should be avoided as the cracks in the wood provide a breeding ground for organisms. Food contamination is illustrated in Fig. 22.

A plentiful supply of hot water and detergent is needed for washing up and as many articles as possible should be rinsed in cold water and left to dry in a covered rack. Tea towels and dishcloths must be washed frequently.

Internal Parasites

Neglect of the elementary rules of food hygiene may lead to the infestation of the intestines by parasitic worms.

Threadworms (*Oxyuris vermicularis*) appear in the stools as small white threads, the eggs having been swallowed with infected food or from unwashed hands. The worms migrate out of the anus at night causing intense irritation and in scratching the hands and fingernails become a vector for the parasite. Treatment consists of administering a drug such as piperazine and the whole family must be treated simultaneously. Ointment can be applied to the anal area to allay irritation and the wearing of gloves at night may help to prevent reinfestation.

Tapeworms (*Taenia saginata* found in beef and *Taenia solium* found in pork) are less common in the UK because of strict regulations concerning meat. All meat should be thoroughly cooked. An infested person may have gastrointestinal upsets and will see segments of worm passed in the stools. Treatment is the administration of oral dichlorophen and careful inspection of stools to check for the excretion of the worm.

Roundworms (*Ascaris lumbricoides*) are also uncommon in Britain. Eggs are taken in with contaminated water or food, and treatment is with a drug such as piperazine.

General Health Measures

Rest

Rest is needed to combat fatigue of which there are two kinds, physical and mental. The amount of rest each individual requires at night can be estimated by his readiness to get up each morning (see p. 51). At the age of 16 years about nine hours' sleep is required and for most adults an average of six to eight is normal. Factors conducive to sound sleep include warmth, comfort, quietness, physical tiredness and freedom from worry. The mattress should be firm but resilient enough to support the spine in a horizontal position. Its springiness should vary with the weight of the person. Bedclothes should be warm but not too heavy. Electric blankets are excellent provided they are used strictly according to the manufacturers' instructions. The bedroom should be warm but not stuffy and there should be free circulation of air. Many people find a walk after supper and a warm bath before going to bed are helpful and relaxing but no physical factors will be effective in producing sleep if the mind is overactive or worried.

Recreation

Recreation is an essential part of the maintenance of health and will relieve mental fatigue and staleness. Most people find work is necessary, not only for the money it brings in, but also to enable them to get some degree of satisfaction and contentment out of life. A person who has a job which he really enjoys doing is particularly fortunate but it is still necessary to give adequate time to recreation which should refresh the mind and restore enthusiasm for life. Hobbies are often taken up to provide an alternative to the normal working life. A person with a sedentary or academic job may enjoy a hobby which is active or which enables him to learn a craft. Another individual whose days are spent in physical tasks may enjoy a hobby which is academic in nature. In either case a contribution is being made to the relaxation which follows the lowering of nervous tension. Holidays also frequently provide a contrast to the normal environment and should be chosen with this in mind. Mental health is also maintained by a breadth of interests and by freedom from stress and worry. Problems should be dealt with as they occur by discussion with friends or by taking professional advice where this is necessary. Once a decision has been made about the action to be followed this should be adhered to and active efforts made to put the problem out of the mind.

Eye Care

Healthy eyes need little care. Using them for reading or watching television will not harm the eyes although overuse may cause general fatigue. If a book must be held too close to be read, the eyes should be tested for shortsightedness and a child who squints should be seen by a doctor.

Exercise and posture

Fresh air and exercise are both important to the mainten-ance of good health and in many cases can conveniently be taken together. A person who is on her feet all day indoors, such as a housewife or a nurse, has more need of fresh air than of exercise while a sedentary worker in an office all day will need both. Exercise stimulates the circulation and ensures good ventilation of the lungs and it also improves muscle tone and increases the appetite thus helping to prevent constipation. Exercise taken in the fresh air has a stimulating effect on both mind and body and mention has already been made of the production of vitamin D by the action of sunlight on skin.

Good posture is important in the maintenance of health and is most likely to be neglected when sitting at a desk or during leisure moments. Desks and chairs should be of the correct height for the individual so that the back is supported and the feet are on the floor. When standing the weight should be distributed evenly and heavy objects should be lifted with a straight back, bending the knees and hips to pick up the object and straightening them to lift it.

A great deal of pain for which no organic cause can be found is due to habits of faulty posture and can be relieved by the correction of these faults. Faulty posture causes pain in the back, at first when the person is tired, later occurring earlier in the day. It is also more common to find strains and sprains of muscles among those who have a faulty posture— later effects include osteoarthritis of joints. Continuing pain causes increased muscular tension which results in increased symptoms. Also a person may eventually become depressed and incapable of dealing with life adequately. Eventually general health will be affected and the sufferer will become easily tired and will have a poor appetite.

Whether sitting or standing the body must be balanced with the vertex held high and the chin 'tucked in' or at least not allowed to poke forward (see Fig. 23). The chest must be wide and the sternum raised with the shoulders relaxed. The muscles of the neck and back must not be stretched or tense; there will be no need for this if the body is balanced and the weight over the balls of the feet as opposed to the knees. Abdominal muscles should be toned and the knee joints balanced with the legs straight.

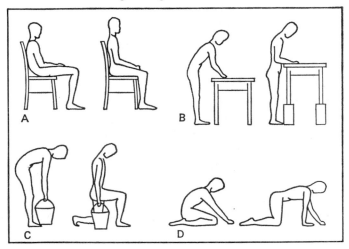

23. The four pairs of figures illustrate the incorrect and correct posture for: A, Sitting on a chair; B, Working at a bench or table; C, Lifting a weight; D, Working in a kneeling position. In each pair the incorrect posture is on the left and the correct on the right.

Clothing

Clothing is worn for protection against heat and cold, for personal adornment and to conform to the moral and ethical standards of the culture to which each individual belongs. It is important that the garments chosen should be easily laundered and should be comfortable. Light coloured clothes are worn in warmer weather because they reflect the sun's rays and help to keep the body cool. Brighter and darker clothes absorb the sun's rays and are therefore warmer in winter. There are many synthetic fabrics available today which wear well and are very easily laundered. The use of these fabrics has done much to raise standards of personal hygiene as they can be washed and dried overnight in many instances, but they are not absorbent and are therefore not very suitable for use in very hot climates.

Shoes

Shoes should be carefully fitted to ensure that they are broad enough and of the right length. Shoes which do not fit well cause corns and callouses which are painful as well as being unsightly and will contribute towards the formation of bunions. Very high heels and thick platform soles cause the weight of the body to be thrown off-balance which is bad for the posture as well as being ugly in appearance and is particularly important in pregnancy (see p. 8).

6

Health Education II

Principles

Health education is concerned with teaching the principles of healthy living. It is one of the methods of preventive medicine and its body of knowledge is drawn from the sciences of medicine, physiology, psychology and sociology. The aims of health education as defined by the World Health Organization are:

(1) *To make health a valued community asset:*
For this to be achieved there must be full development and use of appropriate health services. It is important for each individual to know something of how the health service is organized so that he may make effective use of it and when necessary be critical of its methods.

(2) *To equip people with the knowledge and skills that they can use to solve their health problems:*
Health education seeks to prevent disease, where this is possible, by education and by attempting to influence and modify public attitudes to illness. For example, in the field of mental health the education of lay people about the nature of psychiatric illness and the factors which may predispose

to mental breakdown helps to dispel fear, fosters greater understanding and sympathy towards the mentally ill and eventually leads, it is hoped, to earlier detection of illness and sound progress in treatment and rehabilitation. Similarly, public attitudes concerning cancer, family planning and venereal disease may be modified by correct teaching, thus leading to greater public concern about the need for early detection of malignant disease, the 'population explosion' and the high incidence of gonorrhoea.

(3) *To promote the development of the health service:*
Research into current social problems and changes is necessary to assess specific needs and lead to the provision of a full and adequate health service.

There are nine major areas of health education (Burton 1953):

> Child care
> Mental health
> Prevention of accidents
> Hygiene
> Immunization
> Improvement of doctor–patient relationship
> Nutrition
> Teaching of human biology
> Rehabilitation after illness or injury

Specific teaching in each of these areas aims to educate so that health standards are raised and the individual sees the need for his own response to the situation, if necessary by changing his behaviour.

Health Education in Britain

The earliest examples of health teaching directed towards the individual occur within the family unit. Parents teach their children the basic rules governing personal hygiene, diet, etc., as well as laying down fundamental attitudes to life. Later, when a child enters school his teacher assumes the role of health educator and the child is also influenced by the behaviour of his classmates. Each phase of life presents particular difficulties and appropriate health education is directed towards each vulnerable group. Thus the adolescent may be involved in discussions about sex, smoking or drug-taking organized by medical personnel, church or youth leaders. The expectant mother receives continuous care and counselling throughout pregnancy and childbirth and afterwards while her child is young. Specific health education campaigns concerning topics such as family planning, obesity and the early detection of lung and cervical cancer are aimed at those in the 20 to 50 age group and may be organized in places of employment. The elderly constitute a particularly vulnerable group in society and health education programmes concerning preparation for retirement, the importance of diet and exercise and the social benefits available are geared to their needs (see Chapter 9).

Much of this type of health education goes out in the form of posters and via the mass media of press, radio and television. The presentation of health education material is important and sometimes 'disguise' is necessary for it to be effective. Thus 'pure' health education concerning biology or physiology will have little public appeal but health education put out through radio and television programmes like 'The Archers' or 'General Hospital' command lively interest. Occasionally when a specific campaign is thought to be especially important and relevant to present-day needs, shock tactics may be used, as in the poster issued by the Department of the Environment in Britain (Fig. 24) showing the results of *not* wearing a safety belt.

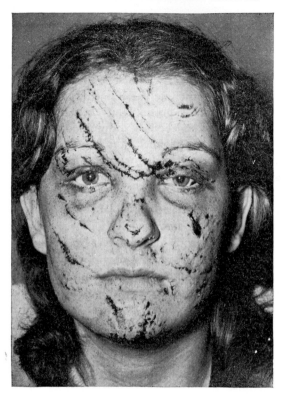

24. A poster, encouraging motorists *and* their passengers to wear safety belts *even* on a short drive.

Health Education under the National Health Service

All workers in the health service are involved to some extent in health education. Doctors, nurses, midwives, health visitors, chiropodists and pharmacists all, during the course of their working day, give counselling and health teaching to individuals or to groups. The Area medical officers, public health inspectors and health visitors are actively engaged in the field of health education, particularly the health visitor whose role is principally that of health educator and adviser. She is involved daily with the person-to-person giving of health education in the home, school and welfare clinic.

From April 1st, 1974, responsibility for the administration of health education rests with the Area Health Authorities but local authorities continue to have the power to carry out health education under Section 179 of the Public Health Act 1936, especially with regard to their responsibilities for environmental health, the control of communicable disease and food poisoning.

The Secretary of State for Health and Social Services has overall responsibility for deciding on policy and developing the health education services but the central department delegates functions to the Health Education Council and to Regional and Area Health Authorities. The Health Education Council was established by the Government in 1968 and is concerned with the planning and promotion of Health Education at national level. The Council mounts national health education campaigns, promotes research and assists the Area Health Authorities with the provision of posters, leaflets, audio-visual aids and exhibition material.

At Area Health Authority level the Area Medical Officer will decide on the priority given to Health Education but many Authorities now employ full-time Health Education Officers. Such officers are usually health service workers (frequently health visitors) who have received special training. Their work involves identifying the needs of the area in which they work and then subsequently planning local health education campaigns. They are also concerned with the organization and supply of Health Education material to health centres, clinics and schools, etc. They may also be responsible for the in-service training in health education given to health service personnel such as doctors, nurses, health visitors and midwives.

At the present time there is a shortage of trained health education officers but courses are being arranged for those wishing to specialize in this field and eventually it is hoped that the health education service will expand and be evenly spread throughout the country.

World Health Organization

Internationally, health education is carried out by the World Health Organization. This was established in 1946 and is responsible for the development of health education in each member state. The organization undertakes research into cultural attitudes and beliefs in order to provide suitable public health programmes in under-developed countries.

Specific topics

Smoking

Smoking presents one of the most common problems in health education because it is still seen by young people as an indication of maturity and because many older people feel a need to continue and increase cigarette consumption in order to relieve tension.

Children of primary school age must be given the facts about the dangers of smoking though at this age they are more likely to be impressed by the likelihood of increased breathlessness interfering with their football prowess than by the serious conditions which may develop in later years. Smoking itself cannot make a boy tough and mature though many adolescent smokers pretend it does. A boy who smokes may be seen by other, wiser children as a failure trying to prove he isn't one, though many weaker children will unfortunately follow his example. The benefits claimed for smoking are grossly exaggerated and the cost is prohibitive, but if parents are tolerant towards smoking and they themselves smoke heavily it will be very difficult to convince children otherwise.

The risks of smoking during pregnancy have already been mentioned in Chapter 1. There is definite evidence of increased risk of spontaneous abortion, premature labour and babies who are very small for their degree of maturity. Of all cases of cancer 25 per cent are found to be suffering from a primary growth in the lung and it is estimated that 1 in 8 of all heavy smokers will die of the condition. The increased number of deaths from cancer of the lung may be in part due to better diagnosis but much of it is due to a real increase in incidence. Men are more often affected than women. The death rate increases with greater cigarette consumption and it must be stressed that it is never too late to give it up.

It is said to be the tar content of cigarettes which is most important as a cause of lung cancer and other respiratory conditions such as bronchitis. The secretion of mucus is stimulated by tobacco smoke which also slows the action of the ciliated lining of the respiratory tract and delays the removal of the secretions.

Nicotine is the substance which may be responsible for an increased incidence of coronary thrombosis among heavy smokers because of its action on heart and blood vessels. It also affects the digestive tract and the kidneys.

Sex Education

Most normal adolescents are interested in and want to discuss the social and emotional relationships which exist between young men and women. They increasingly regard sexual behaviour as a venture in which both partners play an equal part and many approve of premarital intercourse if both partners desire it and when the relationship is a steady one. The dangers of cohabitation with casual acquaintances must be pointed out to them but once they have this information the decision must be left to the individual. Adolescence is a time for the discovery of identity and it is not surprising that this exploration should include sexual relationships. Effective contraception (see Chapter 1) gives the freedom for such exploration but young women in particular should be made aware of the emotional trauma which is associated with casual cohabitation in which satisfaction and fulfilment cannot be found.

Explanation regarding sexual relations should be given in early stages and as interest is aroused and must always be factually correct. Failing this, a child will gain his information from books or friends and be in possession of facts which are incorrect and attitudes which are undesirable. No straight questions should remain unanswered and every youngster should enter adolescence with an adequate factual knowledge of sexual relationships.

It must be understood that fertilization can occur without full intercourse as sperms can be propelled in the vaginal secretions until an area is reached where fertilization is possible. This means that sexual contact, in the absence of intercourse, can result in pregnancy.

The Abortion Act of 1967 was introduced in an effort to reduce the number of illegal abortions with their high mortality. A legal abortion may be carried out if two medical practitioners are of the opinion that the mental or physical health of the mother or her children would be seriously affected if the pregnancy were allowed to continue.

Veneral Disease

The number of cases of venereal disease is increasing, particularly among the young, because of promiscuous sexual intercourse. Better health education of young people in schools and youth clubs is needed urgently to reduce this promiscuity, though results so far have not been encouraging.

Gonorrhoea is the most common venereal disease with 50 000 cases each year. It is contracted only by sexual contact with an infected partner. Three to ten days after infection there is a yellow discharge and the inflammation may also cause discomfort on micturition. Treatment is with penicillin and the cure must be confirmed by follow-up visits. Untreated or inadequately treated disease may cause sterility in both men and women. An infection severe enough to cause chronic salpingitis and resulting sterility may nevertheless be asymptomatic at a time when treatment would be effective.

Syphilis is less common but more dangerous. It is also transmitted during intercourse and if a pregnant woman has the disease the unborn child may also be affected. A child with congenital syphilis is shown in Fig. 25. Following an incubation period of about 25 days a painless ulcer will appear on the sex organs which is highly infectious and will spread if it remains untreated. The second stage is also highly infectious and there is systemic ill health with loss of appetite and weight, and a rash on the body. The third stage is described as the latent stage and lasts for periods varying from several months to a lifetime, during which the infection seems to have disappeared, though it is in fact still highly infectious. In the fourth stage the irreversible damage which has been increasing over the years becomes apparent but by this time treatment can only prevent complications and alleviate symptoms such as deafness, blindness, brain damage, paralysis and insanity, all of which can occur in the untreated patient. Treatment during the early stages of the disease is with penicillin and if treatment is started early for the pregnant woman congenital syphilis in the child may be prevented.

Other infections may occur in the genital tract and a doctor's advice should always be sought.

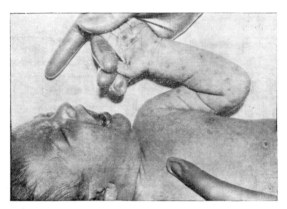

25. Congenital syphilis.

The prevention of venereal disease depends on the complete and efficient diagnosis and treatment of all cases. Special clinics are run for the treatment of these diseases and any person can attend without an appointment and in complete confidence. Specially trained nurses and social workers are employed to trace contacts because examination of cohabiting partners is an important part of prevention. Defaulters must be followed up so that treatment can be completed and complications prevented. Mention has already been made of the importance of health education in avoiding promiscuity and of the routine serological testing of all pregnant women, both of which play a part in the prevention of venereal disease.

Alcohol

As with so many other pleasures alcohol causes no problems if taken in moderate amounts at suitable times. A moderate quantity aids relaxation, enhances enjoyment of social occasions, gives relief from tension and improves a good meal. That it also impairs judgment and slows reaction time is sometimes lost sight of in the euphoria which is produced. The effects of excessive amounts of alcohol may be acute or chronic.

Acute alcohol poisoning is most dangerous when it is combined with driving a vehicle. Before actual drunkenness occurs there is a condition of slowed mental process during which a person may appear to behave normally and his slowed reaction time is not apparent unless it is put to the test in an emergency situation. A concentration of 50 mg alcohol per 100 ml of blood is the highest level which is consistent with safe driving and for many people this figure is reached with the consumption of one pint of beer or two small whiskies, though sensitivity to alcohol varies with the individual and with the time and amount of the last meal. Tranquillizers and sedatives also potentiate the effects of alchohol. Blood alcohol levels reach a peak 30 to 60 minutes after drinking and it takes about two hours for the quantity of alcohol mentioned above to be oxidized. Drunkenness is characterized by behaviour changes, mental confusion and incoordination followed by coma. Vomiting is common in acute alcoholism and may be the reason why death is rare, though when it does occur it is often due to asphyxia from inhaled vomitus.

Chronic alcohol poisoning causes nutritional deficiencies because of loss of appetite due to gastritis. After some years cirrhosis of the liver is a common finding. In addition to the physical effects the alcoholic is in danger of losing his job, with resulting financial deprivation, loss of friends, breakdown of marriage and possible criminal offences connected with obtaining money for the alcohol he needs. Addiction to alcohol is a condition which requires medical and psychosocial therapy in its treatment. The organization known as 'Alcoholics Anonymous' is formed of people who are alcoholics but have learned to deal with their addiction and it can be very helpful to the chronic alcoholic who is really anxious to break from his dependence.

Drugs

Any person who finds it necessary to take any drug regularly to gain relief from any symptom should see a doctor. There is no drug which is entirely free from side effects and none should be taken as a routine without medical supervision. Mention has already been made of the dangers associated with drug taking during pregnancy (Chapter 1) and with the storage of drugs in the home (Chapter 3).

A more serious problem is that of the person, frequently young, who becomes emotionally or physically dependent on drugs. He is often a person who has found difficulty in facing the pressures of every-day life and who may be immature and emotionally inadequate. If at this time he also has access to a supply of one or more drugs, and is in the company of acquaintances who will accept and encourage him in his experimentation the dependence may be initiated. The first feelings are of emotional relief and well-being but as the effects of the drug wear off the insecurity and inability to deal with problems returns only to be relieved by further drug taking in increasing amounts to gain the same effect. Emotional dependence can occur on any tablet or injection, the most important factor being the belief of the taker in the efficacy of the drug. Physical dependence occurs on opiates, sedatives, analgesics, tranquillizers and cerebral depressants and stimulants; a person who is dependent will beg, steal and cause physical harm to others in order to get the drugs he needs.

Drug dependency must be regarded as a progressive condition which leads to cardiac and organic brain disease as well as to personality changes. Families of drug takers are involved because of the hardship inflicted on them by the loss of jobs and financial insecurity until the community is burdened with providing the necessary support.

Drug dependence requires treatment and attempts are made to rehabilitate the addict both mentally and socially. Withdrawal causes muscular pain in arms and legs and violent nausea and vomiting, but these symptoms can be relieved with other drugs. During this withdrawal period help may be accepted which would otherwise be refused.

7

The Adolescent

The word adolescence means 'growing towards maturity' and it is used to describe the period of transition between childhood and adult life.

Physical Health

Physical Development

Adolescence is marked by the onset of puberty and it is at this time that profound physical changes take place which have direct bearing on mental health and development. It is a time of rapid physical growth for both boys and girls, though the difference in progress between the sexes is maintained with girls about two years ahead of boys. The growth spurt in girls reaches its maximum around the age of twelve and is almost over by seventeen. In boys it is at its maximum at about fourteen and has usually ceased by eighteen or nineteen. This rapid development of the long bones may cause loss of coordination in movement and clumsiness is typically a feature of adolescence.

For girls the first apparent body change is an increase in

fat and the widening of the hips. The breasts will begin to enlarge and this will be accompanied by the growth of pubic hair and later of that in the axillae.

In boys voice changes start about the time puberty is reached but may not be completed until a few years later. There is rapid growth of the male sex organs, the testes and the penis, and the pubic hair becomes more dense and shows pigmentation. Later there will be broadening of the chest and shoulders and increasing growth of hair in the axillae and on the trunk, arms, legs and face. The facial proportions also change and the features tend to become more angular.

Puberty. When a girl begins to show the physical changes mentioned above, it is important that careful explanation is given to her so that she is prepared for the onset of the first menstrual period. This is a definite date and is called the menarche but it is only part of the ongoing process of puberty and it does not mean that the girl is fully mature. In Britain the menarche usually occurs about the age of thirteen but there is an ongoing tendency for it to occur earlier and it is not uncommon to find it occurring at eleven years in some children. It can be a profound shock to a child if she experiences the menarche without having been adequately prepared. She should be encouraged to appreciate that menstruation is a sign that she is approaching womanhood and that it is a normal physiological process which will not interfere with normal living. She should be given soft, absorbent pads to use and be taught to change them whenever necessary to prevent chafing and odour. Internal tampons are safe and satisfactory for use by an older girl; when inserted correctly they give rise to no sensation and many women prefer them. All pads and tampons should be wrapped in newspaper and burnt, or may be flushed down the lavatory if they are disposable.

Some women experience discomfort just before and during the first stages of the menstrual period. This discomfort, known as dysmenorrhoea, may be due to retention of fluid and usually disappears shortly after the period begins, but persistent discomfort or pain should be referred to a doctor.

A daily bath or shower is desirable during menstruation or if this is not possible, thorough washing and drying of the vulval area. There are many products on the market which are advertised as being aids to personal freshness for use during menstruation. Most are effective and are pleasant to use but they are expensive and will only be helpful when used in addition to thorough cleanliness. Normal daily exercise can be taken with safety and there is no truth in the old wives' tales that it is not safe to wash the hair, or to paddle, during the period.

Boys, too, should be prepared for the changes which occur at puberty and for the onset of seminal emissions, particularly at night.

Physical Appearance

Because physical growth tends to be erratic during adolescence the young person may both feel and look awkward. Clothes are important in helping to overcome this difficulty and should be chosen by the individual as far as possible. Clothes worn by adolescents are chosen to indicate the gulf they feel between themselves and the older generations. It is important to them, also, to be seen as a member of a group and to this end they wear clothes that are similar to those being worn by everyone else in the same age group.

The tendency among young girls today is not to wear very much make-up though, as with many other fashions, this one will no doubt change overnight. If make-up is to be used at all it should be applied correctly and many schools have lessons in beauty care for older girls. Failing this, a gift voucher for a lesson in beauty care might make a welcome gift for a teenager. Young girls should avoid the standard oily cosmetics and should choose from a medicated range. The foundation should be applied thinly or it may block the pores and encourage oiliness of the skin. Loose face powder is better than a cream powder and the foam puff with which it is applied should be washed frequently.

If the face is spotty, blue-toned lipstick shades should be avoided and also very pale colours which will highlight any red spots. Mid-coral, peach and browny pink shades will make spots seem less prominent. Orange-toned lipsticks should be avoided if the skin is sallow.

Make-up may be removed with a cleansing milk, because it comes off more easily when 'wetted' by oil rather than water, but a cleansing lotion is not sufficient on its own and its application should always be followed with a wash with medicated soap and warm water, followed by a good rinse and thorough drying.

Acne can be a problem during adolescence. Of teenagers, 80 to 90 per cent have some degree of spots, pimples and blackheads on face and shoulders and many of a sufficiently severe degree to cause acute embarrassment. The affected areas should be washed thoroughly three or four times each day using a medicated soap or a prescribed lotion, and then they should be rinsed and dried thoroughly. Face flannels should be boiled twice each week or may be disposable. The skin should not be touched or fingered and scratching should be avoided because it increases the risk of secondary infection. The hair, which tends to be greasy, should be washed frequently as the skin condition may be worse where the hair touches it, e.g. on the forehead. Pillowcases should be changed frequently—on alternate days if possible. For special occasions a flesh-tinted medicated stick may be applied to tone down prominent red areas or pustules. Gradual exposure of the shoulders to sunshine may be beneficial since the ultraviolet rays help to clear acne; fresh air and exercise are also helpful. Stress, excitement and tension all tend to aggravate acne and it may be found to become worse at the time of examinations or when changing jobs and at other times of emotional upset. Reassurance should be given that the situation is only temporary and will revert to normal and that the youngster will eventually grow out of the condition.

Diet

Attention should be paid to the diet and plenty of protein and fresh fruit and vegetables should be included. A pint of milk should be taken daily in addition to plenty of other fluids. For the acne sufferer, pastries and sweets should be avoided and chocolate has been found to aggravate the condition in some people. Apart from these restrictions, adolescents usually have good appetites and because of the growth spurt need a high calorie diet, 2500 to 3000 kilocalories for girls, and 3500 to 3800 for boys, containing plenty of protein. They should be advised against excessive amounts of carbohydrate, which are a great temptation when they are very hungry. A substantial cooked breakfast will help to prevent hunger later in the morning.

Rest and exercise

During adolescence there is a tendency to get overtired very quickly and adequate rest must be ensured. Time must be made for the enjoyment of eating meals at a leisurely pace and for outdoor exercise and recreation.

The most common cause of death in the 15 to 19 age group is

accidents, road accidents forming the highest percentage. Accidents involving motor-cycles account for 30 per cent of deaths from all causes.

Mental Health

The adolescent phase of development is traditionally seen as one of conflict, both with oneself and with the outside world. Western society expects a great deal of young people—the achievement of emotional independence, the completion of sexual identity, the choice of a career, the taking on of social responsibilities and the preparation for marriage—all with minimal guidance. The unfamiliarity of the physical changes which take place, along with the increase in the sex drive, may give rise to major adjustment problems. The adolescent, situated as he is between child and adult, may not know what is expected of him or how he should react to a given situation. Thus there tends to be a loss of emotional stability and a resurgence of preschool behaviour. The adolescent may become rebellious, negative and irrational; like the small child he is testing the reactions of those around him. He needs at this time both to receive and to show tenderness and affection and it is not uncommon to see an adolescent display-ing gentleness towards an animal or a young child. The adolescent also needs to feel that he is an accepted member of a group, to undertake responsibility and to experience adven-ture so that he himself feels that he is approaching adulthood.

Progress towards maturity is a gradual process of the development of independence, which sometimes involves the rejection of previously accepted ideas and values. Parental beliefs may be challenged and great tolerance is needed towards an adolescent during this stage. The best influence remains one of example and reasoning brings greater success than giving an order. It is at this time that the rewards of a free upbringing and of only giving a firm order when it is really necessary can be seen. It may take an adolescent a considerable time to realize that adults have duties and obligations and cannot just please themselves and that these obligations may mean accepting responsibility for others as well as for themselves. There is a great need for the expression of personality by an adolescent in the form of personal possessions and the need for privacy. These needs are best satisfied by the provision of a room for the sole use of the young person but failing this a lockable cupboard may help to satisfy the need. Regular pocket money is important for all children but is essential in adolescence so that a degree of independence can be achieved. It should be made clear exactly what expenditure is to be covered by the weekly allowance so that budgeting can be practised.

Mood swings are common at this age and can be difficult to deal with. Any personal achievement helps adolescents through this negative phase and parents can only offer praise when there is success and sympathy and kindness when there is failure. As it has been throughout childhood the place of the father remains important to the growing girl and boy. There may be many interests in common between a father and his son and when these can be shared, a real companionship develops between them. The relationship between a girl and her father will influence her attitude towards men in general and the happiest relationship develops when a father takes a real interest in his daughter's activities and hobbies. If this interest is accompanied by real companionship and love, the girl will be helped to attain a friendly and confident attitude to the opposite sex.

Intellectual ability develops rapidly during this period and maximum intelligence is usually reached between the ages of 16 and 18. There is a development from concrete to abstract thinking and an awakening of interest in politics, religion and social problems.

Sexual development during adolescence can be seen to have several phases, beginning with the 'gang phase' during which there is natural segregation of the sexes in gang formation. Intense loyalty to the group exists and remnants of this period persist into adult life and are seen as devotion to a particular political party, group activity or to church life. Out of the sense of belonging to a group the need develops for one individual friend, generally of the same sex, with whom one can share confidences. The transition then follows from homosexual friendship to full heterosexuality during which time there may be several 'flirtations' before complete 'falling-in-love' occurs and final choice of a marriage partner is made. Educationally as well as physically the girl matures earlier than the boy. The knowledge that indiscriminate sexual relationships may mean children produces a greater sense of responsibility in an adolescent girl than in a boy of the same age.

The way in which parents react to adolescent behaviour may have far-reaching influence in their child's adjustment to adult life. They need to recognize that the child is growing up and is striving for independence. For some parents this may not be easy. They need to maintain a good relationship with the child by continuing to provide an atmosphere of love and security, by showing interest in the child's activity, offering encouragement and by not making rigid rules which may only result in the sort of parent–child conflict seen in earlier years. Wherever possible parents should avoid offering direct criticism of an adolescent's clothes, hairstyle or opinions since this causes him to feel foolish and tends to give rise to rebellion and resentment, whereas constructive criticism given with gentleness and tact may produce the effect desired by parents. Positive encouragement and support from the immediate family, along with guidance from teachers and others, particularly with regard to preparation for the responsibilities of marriage and parenthood will aid successful growth through adolescence and lead to the development of a mature adult.

Unless both parents and children are prepared for it, adolescence can be a trying time for the whole family. Adults expect adolescents, particularly those who appear physically mature, to behave as adults and are disappointed when they behave as children. Adolescents expect to be treated as adults but frequently behave like children. Youth, inexperience and lack of knowledge are often held against them as a crime and a derisive 'you'll know better when you're older' just aggravates the situation. Being not yet mature enough to 'make allowances', the adolescent who finds his parents are wrong about something may assume they are wrong about most things and when he himself is right he may think he 'knows it all'. Another problem arises when parents, who may not have had the educational opportunities that their child has had, feel they cannot compete with the erudition shown by their offspring.

A problem which has increased in recent years is one of wanton damage by groups of teenagers. The destruction frequently affects half-constructed buildings, empty houses, public buildings such as community centres and schools and telephone booths. It is often planned to some degree by a group or gang and seems in many cases to be engendered by boredom. A harmful pattern of behaviour has been established which is difficult to eradicate; what was labelled naughtiness in children becomes vandalism in adolescents because of their increased physical strength.

Facilities for recreation for all age groups are very important and provide outlets for the abundant energy many young people have. Playing fields and rough areas with trees and streams offer endless scope and indoor athletics are also a good outlet for energy but none of these measures will cure vandalism though they may prevent its occurrence in some cases. Most young people gain support from others of a similar age and must belong to one or many groups where they can be accepted in a variety of roles.

8

The Adult

A considerable amount of attention is paid by various agencies to the health of the young and the old but rather less to that of the adults in the 'in-between' years, from which are drawn most of the leaders of society. Many of the general aspects of the maintenance of health which have been mentioned in connection with children and adolescents are applicable to adults, particularly personal hygiene and the value of a good mixed diet. Some aspects of health care are, however, rather more specific in their application.

General Health Care

Obesity

In Western society obesity is the most common form of malnutrition among adults. Any person who is more than 10 per cent above the normal weight for his or her height and build is described as being obese and the condition develops when the amount of food eaten is greater than the amount of energy expended. Almost any pathological condition is aggravated by obesity but there are some conditions which are more commonly associated with some degree of excessive weight. Statistics show an increased mortality due to hypertension and coronary artery disease and in long-standing obesity there is an increased incidence of diabetes. A continuing high level of blood cholesterol is frequently found in obese people and among such people gall stones are not uncommonly found. The strain of carrying the excess weight is laid mainly on the spine, hips, knees and ankles and these joints may become painful even in the absence of osteo-arthritic changes. Another hazard is the increased occurrence of complications of pregnancy due to obesity. The beneficial effects of weight reduction are shown by a reduced mortality and morbidity and a loss of symptoms such as dyspnoea, indigestion due to hiatus hernia and painful joints due to arthritis.

There are many diet sheets which, if followed closely, will result in loss of weight. For most people a permanent change in eating habits is needed if they are persistently overweight and such a radical change is more effective than the 'crash' diets publicized in magazines. The diet recommended by Dr John Yudkin, Professor of Nutrition at Queen Elizabeth College of the University of London, will achieve both loss of weight and a change in eating habits if adhered to strictly. It is based on a free intake of protein and fat while at the same time restricting carbohydrate. Another helpful fact is that frequent small protein meals are more effective in weight reduction than leaving a long gap between meals so that one is very hungry—which results in eating too much.

Care of the Eyes

It is during adult life, particularly around the age of 40, that some difficulty with vision may commence. Many women notice first that it is no longer easy to thread a needle because they must move it backwards and forwards before they can get it in focus. It is necessary also to hold books farther away than is customary in order to focus on the print. It is advisable to have the eyes tested when this occurs and some authorities recommend that the eyes should be tested at two yearly intervals, rather in the same way that the teeth are checked six-monthly. Eyes should be tested if there is pain or frequent headaches.

No harm can come to the eyes simply by using them, watching television or reading in bed will not damage the eyes in any way. Adequate lighting for any close work will reduce fatigue and there should be a light on in some part of the room while watching television as to watch it in the dark is more tiring. Eye lotions should only be used as and when prescribed; the normal eye does not require artificial irrigation as it is kept moist by the tears which continually flow across the surface of the eye. Ordinary sunshine will not damage the eyes and in normal sunny conditions sunglasses are not necessary. They are helpful when climbing mountains, in snow, in the desert and when sailing or in any situation where there is excessive glare, but the rule is to wear them only for comfort. If glasses are prescribed they should be worn as directed and it is an offence not to wear glasses while driving if one is required to.

Dental Care

The principles of care for adults remains the same as for children. The incidence of dental decay tends to decrease with advancing years, but there is an increased likelihood of difficulties resulting from receding gums. The importance of regular cleaning cannot be overstressed, both by correct and frequent use of the toothbrush and by eating of fibrous foods. Some authorities advocate the use of toothpaste containing fluoride as an adjunct to the prevention of decay. For the arthritic or handicapped person an electric or battery-operated toothbrush may be helpful.

Mental Health

The middle years are a time of maturity and fulfilment when an individual's powers and limitations should be both understood and accepted if happiness and contentment are to be enjoyed. There are however certain areas of stress common to many individuals and it is the coming to terms with these problems which denotes maturity in its fullest sense.

For many adults their work provides a situation in which they may find a sense of purpose and achievement, though many spend their working lives doing a job for which they are not suited. It is hoped that with the fuller provision of vocational guidance services more people will be enabled to find jobs for which they are suited both temperamentally and academically. As the working week becomes shorter more guidance is needed in the use of leisure.

During adolescence the attraction of the opposite sexes is predominantly physical. With increasing age companionship and mutual respect are added to physical attraction and an ability develops to adapt outlook and habits to fit in with those of the marriage partner, though an individual's personality does not change nor should it be expected to. Voluntary organizations such as the marriage guidance council are available to advise on problems which may arise.

The responsibilities of parenthood constitute one of the greatest adaptations which have to be made during adult life. The problems have already been mentioned at some length in previous chapters. It is important that the family should be brought together as a unit when a new baby is born, and that the father and any other children should not be shut out in the consuming mutual dependence of mother and baby.

Bereavement is a situation which may have to be faced at any time but which not uncommonly occurs for the first time during adulthood when the parents of an adult may die. The grief may be less severe for a married person who can share emotions with the marriage partner. In any case grief is natural and should be expressed so that the bereaved can learn to live with the reality of the situation. It is common for a bereaved person to feel remorse about things they might have done for the individual who has died and the knowledge that this is a normal sentiment helps to put it in perspective. It is helpful too if there are practical needs of other people that have to be met so that the bereaved person is helped to realize that life must go on.

Adjustments have to be made continually with increasing years but both men and women become less flexible and tend to become set in their ways. The process of growing older is hindered if behaviour and attitudes appropriate to a younger age group persist; there must be continued growth of personality.

A woman may regret the fact that her children are grown up and no longer need her in the same way. She may react by being overpossessive or by hysterical or depressive behaviour. This may be a problem during the menopause when the physical ability to bear children ceases and a woman may feel that her role of motherhood is finished. She may then feel 'useless', unattractive and lacking in self-confidence and will consequently find it very difficult to go out and make new friends. This period may serve to highlight pre-existing problems in marriage and sexual life and the skilled help of a marriage guidance counsellor may be needed.

A man too may be beginning to feel his age acutely. He becomes aware of failing physical and mental abilities and decline in sexual feeling may give rise to fears of impotence, a problem he may seek to solve by heavy drinking or by searching for relationships with younger women. Also, a man at this time may be at the most demanding stage of his career. He may be realizing the limits of his capabilities, may feel himself a failure or may fear rejection in favour of a younger man. If he is successful he may be under continual work pressure. All these problems will affect the quality of family life.

The prevailing attitude, during this period of life, needs to be one of acceptance, a coming to terms with oneself, one's partner and one's own capabilities and limitations. It should be a time for cultivating interests and hobbies and for participating in the wider concerns of society by involvement in such activities as voluntary work, church councils, etc., where the wisdom of maturity is a valuable asset.

The Menopause

The term menopause describes the end of the reproductive years of a woman and it is colloquially called the 'change of life'. As with puberty, the menopause does not occur overnight, and is in fact a process drawn out over some years in most cases. It can occur any time between the ages of 40 and 55 with an average age of around 50. It is unfortunate that rumour tells of mental stress, flagging energy, obesity, changed appearance, usually for the worse, a decrease in sexual desire and capacity and hot flushes. Some of these symptoms do occur but many are coincident with and not due to the menopause.

The actual pattern of the cessation of menstruation varies considerably, some women having irregular periods for some months before they finally cease, others experiencing a lessening of the flow or a lengthening of the cycle, or both.

What is important is that frequent irregular bleeding is not usual and should be reported to a doctor without delay. The apparent increase in the incidence of cancer of the genital organs at the menopause is due to the expected irregularity causing little notice to be taken of the appearance of frequent small bleeds, known as 'spotting' which is an early and important sign of cancer. By the time this sign is reported to a doctor the condition may be advanced and require extensive treatment.

Hot flushes are a common symptom at the menopause and occur in some degree in 62 per cent of women. They are due to a hormonal imbalance and vary from a mild degree of warmth and blushing to a totally incapacitating flushing of the body with excessive sweating which is not compatible with a normal social life. Some women are unaware that the condition can be treated effectively and easily and may endure it for months or even years unnecessarily.

The hormonal imbalance mentioned above may also be responsible for the mood changes which occur in some women. The feelings suffered are described as sensitivity, irritation, inadequacy and depression. The menopause itself does not cause mental illness but a tendency to this kind of illness may be aggravated at this time. Another contributing factor may be that the family is now grown up and has left home and the housework and cooking have been reduced to a fine art by years of experience and practice. For many people encouragement to take on some activity which is interesting but which she has been too busy to be involved with in the past will resolve the problem.

Occupational Health Service

Occupational health services are concerned mainly with the prevention of disease among employees. The personnel of such a service study the special hazards and problems facing the workers in a particular industry, including the stresses and strains. They are also interested in the environment and conditions in which people work and the human relationships within industry. Another important function is the rehabilitation of sick and injured workers so that they can return to their old jobs or be trained for others more suitable.

The Department of Employment and Productivity maintains a factory inspectorate which has a medical branch and close liaison is also maintained with the Department of Health and Social Security. The Medical Inspectors of Factories are responsible for the investigation of cases of industrial disease and for the inspection of factories from the health aspect. They also supervise the work of the factory doctors who are frequently local general practitioners. All young people under 18 are examined when they start work and periodical examinations are carried out of those who are engaged in dangerous industrial processes.

The medical officer checks on the general cleanliness of the premises, over-crowding, temperature, which must be not less than 15°C (60°F) for sedentary workers, ventilation, lighting, drainage, noise and the provision of adequate lavatory and washing accommodation for both men and women. There are many special regulations made under the Factories Act 1961 concerning the health of workers in particular trades. Examples of these are precautions against anthrax in industries handling animal skins and hides and against lead poisoning in the manufacture of paint and other processes involving lead.

Many large firms have well organized occupational health services with medical and dental surgeries, first aid facilities and full-time staff. In other cases smaller firms have joined forces to provide a similar service from which all their employees can benefit. A major factor in occupational health is good selection so that people are fit to do the job for which they are employed. A person who is liable to dermatitis should not be employed in handling toxic metals and dusts while another person may be psychologically unsuited to the strains and stresses of a certain job. Colour blindness may be a bar to some employment like flying aeroplanes; here also physical fitness is so important that frequent medical examinations are vital.

Employees who are repeatedly absent are usually seen by the doctor. Deterioration in the health of an individual will show as lowered efficiency, increased sickness and absenteeism, general irritability and lowered morale with an increased tendency to accidents. This combination of factors is known as 'occupational fatigue' and may sometimes be due to poor working conditions.

Insurance against industrial injuries is compulsory for practically all employees in Britain. Certain prescribed diseases are described as industrial diseases and the same benefits and conditions apply to these as to industrial injuries. Examples of these diseases are conditions of the respiratory tract in workers in mines, quarries, asbestos works, and the cotton industry. Toxic substances may produce skin lesions such as dermatitis and epithelioma following exposure to oil and tool-setters and similar workers, whose job involves bending over machines with resultant continuous friction and oil contamination, are at risk.

Following industrial injury or sickness most people are able to return to ordinary employment if their jobs are carefully chosen but industrial rehabilitation may be needed to prepare them for a normal day's work and to determine the type of work for which they are best suited. There are 25 industrial rehabilitation units with a total of more than 2000 places. In industrial areas the units are situated within daily travelling distance or residential or hostel accommodation may be made available. Each course is planned individually and is tailored to fit the needs of each person attending. The length of stay varies from two weeks to six months with an average stay of two months. In an industrial atmosphere the disabled person is able to adjust to working conditions and simultaneously remedial treatment helps to build up confidence. Vocational assessment and guidance is an essential feature of each course and training in a skilled trade may follow the rehabilitation course.

Services for the Handicapped

Under the Local Authority Social Services Act 1970 the responsibility for welfare services for the handicapped passed to the Social Service Departments. The aim of all services is to enable the handicapped person to lead as full and independent a life as possible. To this end adaptations to the home may be made to enable wheelchairs to be freely mobile; this may include ramps to replace steps and widening of doorways. A wide variety of equipment may be made available on loan, ranging from large items such as hoists and handrails through alarm devices and entry phones to kitchen accessories. A severely handicapped person may be entitled to financial help with the installation and rental of a telephone, but not with payment for calls. Advice and help for the disabled may be obtained from the Central Council for the Disabled.

Handicapped people may attend day centres or go on outings or weekends with the help of specially equipped buses which have hydraulically operated tail lifts. At the day centres there are recreational facilities and opportunities to learn a craft as well as to meet other people. Help may be given with the provision of television and radio sets and licence payments. Many local authorities and voluntary organizations combine to provide holidays for those who cannot otherwise go away. An attendance allowance is payable for a severely disabled person who requires constant attendance throughout day and night. A library service is available for the housebound and a full laundry service where incontinence is a problem. The services mentioned above are a few of those available, though not every local authority provides the same range of services.

The services available for the physically handicapped are also available to those suffering from mental disorders. Community services for the mentally ill include the provision of day centres which provide rehabilitation programmes for those who will be able to return to work and sheltered employment or occupation for those suffering from chronic mental illness. Hostels provide short-stay accommodation for those not yet ready to return fully to the community and long-stay care for those unable to maintain an independent existence.

An obligation is laid on all employers of not less than 20 persons to employ a quota of registered disabled people—at present 3 per cent of their total employees. The occupations of car park attendant and passenger lift attendant have so far been reserved for the disabled.

9

The Elderly

The improvement in maternal and child health has coincided with an increase in the percentage of elderly people in the population. There is little that can be done at present to prevent the degenerative diseases of old age so the pattern of ill health has changed and chronic disease in an ageing population is more common. The life expectancy of a woman is greater than that of a man by about six years but of these elderly women, 96 per cent are living in their own homes with varying degrees of support and only about 4 per cent require hospital or residential care.

The disappearance of the 'extended family' from urban industrial society presents that society with problems regarding the care of an increasing number of elderly people. The extended family is one in which several generations live close to one another and give mutual support in times of crisis, illness, infirmity and old age. It is still common in rural settings among non-industrialized communities and in countries such as Japan, China and some Mediterranean countries.

In Western society the young are no longer economically dependent on their elders and marriages are not 'arranged' so the young wife is not subservient to the mother-in-law.

Increasing numbers of women go out to work and better transport and expanding opportunities encourage families to disperse. It is increasingly difficult to find someone to look after the elderly in their homes so there is a tendency for the parents to move around the family.

The success of having three generations living together in the same house is dependent to some extent on the size of the house itself. If there is room for separate accommodation for the elderly persons so that they are independent but can call on help if necessary, the plan will work well. It is less likely to work successfully in small overcrowded houses where children may have to move out of bedrooms and there is risk of disagreement between in-laws.

Individual Ageing

As an individual gets older there is progressive loss of vigour and a diminishing ability to adapt to changes in the environment. It becomes more difficult to learn new principles and the elderly person becomes increasingly dependent on habits of behaviour and on long-term memory. There is a gradual decline in the functions of organs until they are only able to maintain life at a slower pace and with reduced reserves.

Mortality and Morbidity

Over the age of 50 the most common causes of death are heart disease, malignancy and respiratory disorders, though in old age there is rarely one single cause of death. In Britain chronic bronchitis accounts for a high percentage of deaths in the elderly.

The chief causes of disability are cardiovascular and respiratory disease, disorders of the locomotor system and of the special senses and symptoms stemming from genitourinary disorders. Some degree of atherosclerosis is normal in the elderly and a raised blood pressure is physiological among European nations. All people over 70 show decreased cardiac efficiency. Those who are subject to chronic bronchitis may attend special clinics where they can receive vaccination against influenza at the beginning of the winter months, can be instructed about correct methods of breathing and be given antibiotic drugs which can be taken at the onset of infection. Tuberculosis is becoming more of a problem among the elderly because treatment is keeping alive many who would have died in earlier years. Rheumatoid and osteo-arthritis can cause severe crippling and defects of legs and feet are common. Proper care, hygiene, adequate exercise and chiropody services are essential in keeping an old person mobile. Deteriorating vision and hearing will cause difficulty in communication and loss of enjoyment of reading, listening to the radio and watching television. Symptoms of genito-urinary disorder such as dysuria, frequency, urgency and nocturia cause social isolation, restrict movement and are a burden on relatives.

Planning for Retirement

Many people who have coped successfully with old age have planned carefully for their retirement. This frequently presents a greater problem for a man than for a woman, who still has shopping, cooking and housework to do, but for any person who leads an active life, successful retirement needs careful preparation. Many local organizations run short courses for people who are soon due to retire and the best time to take such a course is some two to three years before the date of retirement so that there is time to put the new ideas into practice. An important aspect of retirement is the maintenance of a sense of purpose and interest and if this can be channelled into the provision of service for others the feeling of being needed will also be beneficial. In any event, the creation of a wide field of interests in pre-retirement years to which time can be devoted after retirement may give an individual a new lease of life.

General Health Care

Bearing in mind that as age increases body function becomes less efficient, measures to maintain health in the elderly should be aimed at maintaining body function at its optimum, but because the ageing process occurs at a different speed in every individual, no hard and fast rules can be laid down. Exercise and activity should be continued for as long as possible and graded to suit the capability of each individual but at the same time adequate rest is essential, though it should be remembered that the amount of sleep required by the elderly tends to be less than in earlier years. Elderly people feel cold more easily than the young and clothing must be adequate for their needs. Draughts should be avoided and the provision of insulation in houses and of good quality curtains will help in the maintenance of living temperatures at about 20°C (70°F). The defective temperature regulating system in the elderly may result in *hypothermia* in which the body temperature drops far below normal. The old person becomes lethargic and confused with indistinct speech and a tendency to fall. The muscles become rigid and the entire body feels cold to the touch. This condition constitutes a medical emergency and medical aid must be sought. In the meantime the person should be wrapped in blankets in a warm room and given a warm drink. External heat should not be applied in the form of hot water bottles.

Diet. The diet of the elderly is one of the most important factors affecting their health. An adequate daily intake of protein and fresh fruit and vegetables and a total of 9 to 10 cups of various fluids should be taken every day. For a variety of reasons, including cost, adequate amounts of protein may not be consumed but replaced by various forms of carbohydrate. Factors which militate against adequate diet are a possible inability to go shopping, apathy which precludes the cooking of proper meals, loss of appetite, ill-fitting or lack of dentures so that mastication is difficult or even a physiological inability to utilize the food properly. Because of this, anaemia is not uncommon among the elderly. Because the sense of taste is often altered, prepared foods should be tasty and additional seasoning is frequently required. The provision of luncheon clubs, where main meals can be provided at a reasonable cost, helps to overcome this problem for the more active pensioner and gives the additional benefits of social contact, exercise and an outing. For the housebound the 'meals-on-wheels' service provides a main meal three times a week, or more often if required, for a small payment. The responsibility for the preparation of the meals rests with the local authority and the Women's Royal Voluntary Service helps with the distribution. In some areas a delivery takes place in the late afternoon as well as at lunchtime so that more people may benefit from the service.

Deteriorating vision is a common cause of distress and of social isolation in the elderly. Anyone with a history of rapid failure of sight necessitating frequent change of spectacles, or a complaint that vision is better in a dim room than in a bright light, should be investigated by an ophthalmic surgeon.

In some areas routine screening of elderly people for minor health defects is a service provided by the local authority and may help to prevent the multiple pathology which is commonly found on admission to hospital. A routine examination as part of a pre-retirement counselling programme is carried out in some areas.

Mental Health

The maintenance of physical health is an important part of the maintenance of mental health but it is important too that elderly people should have continuing human contact and something useful to do. Without social intercourse and conversation there is deterioration of vocabulary and of mental processes, and progressive deafness leads to isolation unless active measures are taken to combat this. Familiar surroundings are important in preventing mental deterioration and everyone, no matter what their age, needs affection and to be wanted. Independence and the sense of security which comes from sufficient food, warmth and shelter are harder to satisfy in old age and an additional problem is the isolation which is due to having outlived family and friends and to having difficulty in making new friendships as age increases. Some lonely pensioners are helped by encouragement to join a club or to attend a social centre where classes in a variety of subjects are available at a nominal sum. Many voluntary organizations provide social facilities and various forms of craft work in day centres. Another important aspect of the prevention of mental illness is careful and repeated explanation of the social and economic entitlements of the individual and attention to the solving of problems connected with these rights and privileges.

One of the signs of maturity is increased control of feelings and the inhibition of emotional extremes. Older people tend to be less inhibited in their behaviour and feelings are more easily aroused, resulting in outbursts of anger, gratitude or affection in response to events which are themselves trivial. This decline in control combined with forgetfulness may sometimes result in a deterioration in personal habits, particularly in those who live alone. The restrictions on activity and self-sufficiency which are common in old age are not always accepted with good grace and irritability, depression or suspicion may be forerunners to withdrawal of interest from the outside world and increasing self-preoccupation. These facets of personality are often the result of lack of interest by society and are avoided in those who are wanted and loved and feel themselves to be valued and useful.

Old age is often a time when religious feelings are strengthened and those who regard death as a new beginning can anticipate it with serenity. Those who lack religious faith may obtain comfort from their feeling of having lived a useful and purposeful life. Their faith is also a great comfort when elderly people are faced with bereavement. After an initial period of grieving they must be helped to resolve the social, economic and personal problems which confront them and to adapt gradually to the new situation in which they find themselves.

Medical Services

Several of these services have been mentioned already in the appropriate context. Chiropody is most important in keeping an elderly person mobile in comfort and many elderly people cannot attend to their own feet because of stiff knees and hips, shaky hands or failing eyesight or a combination of these disabilities. In most areas there are foot clinics which may be attended free of charge by the elderly or home visits can be arranged for the housebound, though benefit is gained from an outing for whatever reason. In some areas treatment may be arranged privately and the cost met by the local authority. Regular treatment at intervals of six to eight weeks is essential. A home nursing service is available during illness and the district nurse may call to give injections, blanket baths and other purely nursing services. Laundry may be dealt with in some cases and this is particularly valuable where incontinence is a problem. In some areas a night sitter service enables continuous care to be given at night to patients who are ill at home, often where the illness is terminal.

Social Services

There are many social services to which the elderly are entitled. The ones mentioned here are those directly connected with the maintenance of health. The home help service is one which is particularly valuable to the pensioner living alone and unable to look after the home. The home help, who is frequently a married woman, will attend two or three times a week for three to four hours at a time and will assist with routine jobs such as housework, shopping and cooking. The charge for such help is on a sliding scale and many pensioners have the service free. Meals-on-wheels and luncheon clubs have already been mentioned in connection with nutrition. Another valuable service often organized by voluntary associations, is the provision of social clubs and handicraft centres, where the elderly can meet other people, develop an interest in craft work and benefit from the outing. Day care centres are intended to care for elderly people who would otherwise be in hospital. The old person is collected by special transport in the morning and returned home in the late afternoon and during the day will receive all the care which is needed including meals, physiotherapy, occupational therapy and when necessary, such services as hairdressing, bathing and chiropody.

Pensioners who have a supplementary pension are entitled to help with the cost of glasses, dentures, dental treatment, wigs and fabric supports when these are prescribed under the National Health Service and will also receive all medicines on prescription *free of charge*. Surgical appliances are on loan when these are necessary. When it is necessary financial help can be given with the cost of fuel for heating the home; mention has already been made of the dangers of excessive cold in the elderly (see p. 122). Some local authorities help with the cost of holidays for the elderly and many seaside resorts cooperate by making accommodation available at cheap rates at the beginning and end of the summer season.

It is the responsibility of local authorities to provide accommodation for all who need care and attention, regardless of their financial circumstances. A resident would pay what he can, over and above a nominal sum retained for pocket money. Privately run homes must be registered. An elderly person who is unable to care for himself and who is not being adequately cared for by others may if necessary be removed to a suitable hospital on a court order.

Voluntary Organizations

As mentioned previously, there are many voluntary organizations which provide services for the elderly. Such a voluntary service is the 'Good Neighbour' visiting scheme under which elderly people are visited regularly at a mutually convenient time and services such as shopping, changing library books, window cleaning and hairdressing may be undertaken.

Accident Prevention

An important part of the health education of the elderly is concerned with the prevention of accidents (see Fig. 26). Sixty-five of every hundred accidents which occur in the home are to those aged over 65 years and the most common accidents are falls, poisoning and burns and scalds. Good lighting is important in the prevention of falls, particularly on stairways. Frayed carpets, slip mats and trailing flexes may all cause the elderly person to trip; bedroom slippers and 'run over' shoes are also dangerous as one must shuffle in order to keep them on. Any grease or water spilled on the floor should be wiped up immediately. With increasing age greater dependence is placed on vision for maintaining balance,

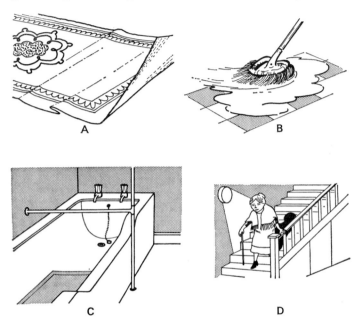

26. A, Loose mats are dangerous particularly on polished floors; B, Spilt water should be mopped up immediately; C, A handrail is helpful in the bathroom; D, Stairways must be lighted.

so there should always be a torch by the bed for use when getting up in the night and a landing light should be put on. Special care is required on stairs, particularly by those wearing bifocal glasses, and handrails should be available, but it must be remembered that in order to make full use of them the hands must be free. Particular care is needed in the bathroom where slipping is common. A vertical handrail by the bath

is a great help to many. An elderly person should be encouraged to hold onto something firm when stooping or reach-
ing to pick things up. Falls are often associated with attacks
of vertigo and with deafness, failing vision and muscular
weakness. Less force is required to fracture a bone in the
elderly because of lack of muscle tone and osteoporosis.

All medicines in the home should be clearly labelled and
safely stored if accidental poisoning is to be avoided. Sleeping
tablets should not be kept by the bed so that a second dose
cannot be taken in error.

Material used for clothing should be of a non-flammable
type and fires should be guarded. All gas and electric fires
have a metal guard fixed to the apparatus but open fires
are particularly dangerous and should have a secure guard in
front. Paraffin heaters are dangerous, particularly the drip-
feed type and their use by elderly people should be dis-
couraged to hold on to something firm when stooping orreach
burns are caused easily when the skin is less sensitive. In the
kitchen, shelves and cupboards should be accessible without
standing on steps or stools and self-lighting gas taps are safer
than those which require manual lighting.

Impaired hearing, particularly for high frequencies, may
be the cause of road traffic accidents as the sound of oncoming
traffic or of horns may be misjudged.

COMMUNITY HEALTH

10

The Home

One of the indications of civilized society is a high standard of housing and a government which legislates for space and light to be a right for all.

Housing

When a new housing development is being planned stress is placed on the importance of broad streets to enable traffic to move safely and wide pavements so that pedestrians can walk about with comfort. Trees set at the pavement edge make a street look more pleasant and give an impression of separation of traffic and pedestrians. They also help to reduce noise. Where space allows, houses and flats may be built round a central area with grass and trees or may be set back from the road with space for a front garden which helps to reduce the noise of traffic. Tall blocks of flats must be built sufficiently far apart so that there is adequate light and ventilation between the blocks and the public buildings, the main shopping centre and places of entertainment should be sited centrally with adequate car parking facilities and public transport.

These important public facilities and services together with community centres, health centres, libraries, churches and play areas and parks must be built as the houses are built for they are essential for the welding together of a community, always a difficulty when all the residents are new to the area. Recreational facilities must also be provided by the local authorities so that there are adequate playing fields and swimming pools for all age groups, and playgrounds for younger children. Homes for 10 000 to 15 000 people are often grouped together within a 'green belt' of undeveloped land so that open space is easily accessible. Such a residential area would be near suitable industry so that residents do not have to travel long distances to work and factories and other industrial premises are frequently confined to an industrial estate so that the noise and traffic are kept away from residential areas.

New towns are built for those people from slum clearance areas who cannot be rehoused in the existing town because of overcrowding. Such groups are often referred to as 'overspill populations' and many have been rehoused in places such as Cumbernauld in Scotland and Skelmersdale in Lancashire. Each of these towns has a population of about 70 000 to 80 000 and traffic and pedestrians have been separated to make residential areas safer for the residents.

One great disadvantage of new towns is the tendency for the entire town to be populated by younger married couples and their children. The young wife is separated from her own family and her old associations and her mother or other older relatives are not easily available for advice or for 'baby sitting' when needed. The result of this may be bewilderment and loneliness which is difficult to overcome. One requirement which has been recognized and fulfilled is the 'corner shop' which not only provides basic necessities but also serves as a meeting place and fulfils a social need.

In 1969, the number of flats throughout Britain was nearing

400 000, a figure likely to go on increasing as the need for more housing continues. A small block of modern flats is shown in Fig. 27. Many flats are in tower blocks (Fig. 28) which present their own problems. The effects of 'high rise' living are many and are not confined to a single social group.

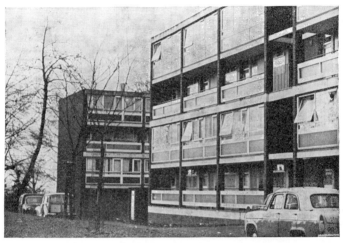

27. A neat and open style for modern flats.

Loneliness and a sense of isolation are probably the most important factors, affecting particularly the mothers of young families who no longer meet for a chat over the garden fence as their grandmothers may have done. Equally the isolation of the elderly and infirm is aggravated and they may feel imprisoned in their 'box' far above ground level, unable to watch and be part of street activity. The sense of community spirit is also lost, especially in those tower blocks built in redevelopment areas which may rehouse families from outside the immediate surrounding area.

The group most likely to suffer from living in high-rise

blocks is preschool children, especially those in large families having other social problems. Research findings collected by the National Children's Bureau have shown that preschool children suffer from a sense of isolation and lack stimulation and the opportunity for mixing with other children. Physical

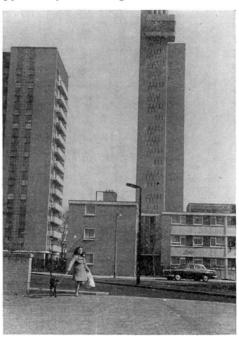

28. High-rise flats.

activity is of necessity restricted by space and this may produce retardation in the development of certain neuromuscular skills, e.g. that needed for climbing stairs. Lack of opportunity for noisy and messy play may also interfere with normal personality development, and other studies have shown that children reared in flats fail to develop fully the ability to explore and experiment. The problems of raising young children in high rise flats may place untold pressures on a young harassed mother and may predispose to 'battering' of the children, to depression and other forms of mental breakdown.

There are certain minimum requirements for satisfactory housing which must be fulfilled if the residents are to be able to live a comfortable and healthy domestic life. The building must be in good repair so that the rooms are dry and there must be proper lighting and ventilation in each room. An inside water supply must be adequate for all needs and is an essential preliminary to the provision of a hot water supply. There should be an inside lavatory and a fixed bath and suitable arrangements for the disposal of waste water and drainage.

Some authorities advocate the siting of lavatory and bath in the same room, particularly where there are children. If this is the case there should be a second lavatory with a small handbasin.

There should be adequate points for artificial lighting and facilities for heating each room. There must be adequate facilities for the preparation and cooking of food and a suitably ventilated larder, though this need has been super-seded in many cases by the provision of a refrigerator. If fuel is to be stored there must be a safe place to store it, and a garage and an out-building suitable for storage of large items such as prams, bicycles and garden tools, add much to comfort and convenience inside the house. A sink in the kitchen is indispensable for most domestic purposes including household washing. Some modern blocks of flats have a communal laundry between a certain number of households. Where the drying of wet clothes is a problem many make use of the 'tumble-dryers' in commercial launderettes.

In temperate climates the living-rooms are usually built facing the sun and the kitchen and bedrooms facing away.

Windows should be large and occupy up to one-third of the wall space. Adequate cupboard and storage space is very helpful and a cupboard which contains the hot water tank and can be used for airing clothes is useful, particularly in the winter months.

A house should offer sufficient space for family activities over and above housework and cooking. Privacy should be available for homework and leisure activities and for a variety of occupations to be carried on simultaneously without interference. Where there are young children, playing space and warmth are required indoors and a safe playing space out of doors. Older children need some space, however small, that they can call their own even if it is only a cupboard, though later they really need a room.

For those homes which do not have the standard amenities a 'House Improvement Grant' may be obtained from the local authority. Up to half the cost, to a predetermined maximum, may be claimed to help with the installation of such items as a lavatory, a fixed bath or shower, handbasin, kitchen sink, hot and cold water supply and adequate heating and lighting.

The Effects of Housing on Health

It is undeniable that those who live in slum areas have poorer health than those who live in good residential districts (Fig. 27). Among the less well housed there is a higher incidence of infectious disease and a greater frequency of complications. Airborne infections such as tuberculosis are more easily spread in overcrowded conditions and more buildings are found to be verminous. The dampness which is caused by defective roofs and gutters and 'rising damp' leads to an increase in rheumatic conditions, increased child mortality and the increased occurrence of chest conditions such as bronchitis in the elderly. Poor housing (Fig. 29) is a contributory factor in the cause of mental illness it prevents the development of normal family relationships. Children cannot work properly and individual pursuits cannot be followed in rooms that are damp, overcrowded, badly lit or cold. In many cases there is a vicious downward spiral of poverty, ill health and ignorance

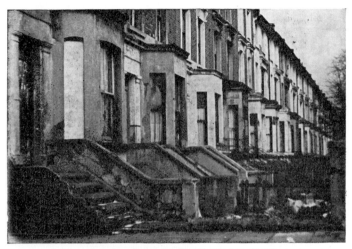

29. An old housing development that has become a slum.

which lead to poor housing, physical and mental ill health which prevent people from coping with a normal working life and leads to greater poverty which in turn leads to more ill health. The local authority can serve a notice on a landlord requiring such repairs to be carried out as are necessary to maintain the health of the occupants.

Infestation. One of the most common effects of poor housing is an increase in the amount of infestation which occurs. Mention has already been made in Chapter 5 of some of the parasites which infest the human body. Old houses are likely to be infested with *bed bugs (Cimex lectularis* see Fig. 30). These are reddish brown in colour and create a characteristic musty odour in a building. They live in walls and furniture, cracks and skirting boards from which they migrate at night to bite humans sleeping in the house. The bites are extremely irritating but in Britain the bugs do not carry other diseases.

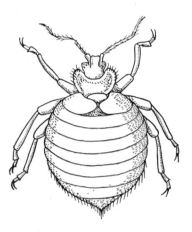

30. Bed bug.

Infested property is very difficult to deal with and must be dealt with by the disinfestation service of the local authority. During rehousing programmes old furniture may be moved in a van which can be sealed so that the contents can be fumigated *en route* to the new premises. The bugs can exist for months without a meal so uninhabited property is as much a risk as any other. The difficulty of moving furniture in overcrowded rooms makes thorough cleaning impossible, but cleanliness, sunlight and fresh air are the best preventive measures.

House flies (Mustica domestica see Fig.3A) do not carry infectious diseases but may spread faecalborne diseases on their legs. After alighting on food, flies and bluebottles regurgitate saliva and defaecate before eating, thus contaminating food further. Flies are controlled by ensuring that compost heaps are as far from the house as possible as flies breed in rotting vegetable matter. Dustbins should always be covered with a tightly fitting lid and food should be covered at all times to

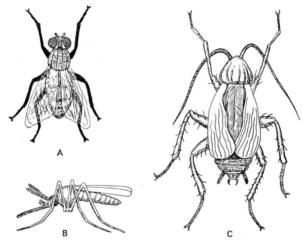

31. A, Housefly; B, Mosquito; C, Cockroach.

prevent contamination, and kept in the refrigerator if possible. Insecticides are used where the problem is a severe one. As with most insects, thorough spring cleaning is one of the best preventive measures that can be taken.

Mosquitoes (*Culex pipiens* see Fig. 31B) are less of a problem in Britain. Though the bites can be very irritating, the insects do not carry malaria, yellow fever or other diseases as they do in tropical countries. Control of mosquitoes depends on the adequate draining of marshland, use of DDT sprays, mosquito proofing of houses and the treatment of aeroplanes to prevent the carrying of infected mosquitoes from a yellow fever zone.

Rats are not uncommon in Britain and can carry a variety of diseases, of which plague is the best known. Though it does not occur in this country continuous precautions are taken at ports to prevent infected rats leaving ships which have come from an area where plague is endemic. The brown rat (*Rattus norvegicus*) is the most common and tends to live at ground level or in burrows and sewers. Routine destruction of rats is carried out in sewers and drains, and all buildings where food is stored must be ratproof. Where rats or mice are suspected the Rodent Officer of the local authority should be called in.

Multiple Occupation

Many problems are created when several families share one house, with perhaps only one room per family and inadequate toilet, washing and cooking facilities for the number of occupants. Local authorities have power to control this problem and to insist on adequate lighting, water supplies, sanitary facilities and heating and sufficient room for the preparation and cooking of food.

Unsatisfactory tenants present a problem in some areas, frequently those designated as slum clearance estates. Many families who are rehoused in modern accommodation need support and guidance in the first few months after the move until they become used to the change. For some the problem is even greater and there may be difficulty in planning ahead budgeting and in looking after their own affairs. If sufficient help is not given the children may be physically neglected and dirty, ill-nourished and backward though the family may be reasonably happy and cruelty uncommon. In other cases there may be drunkenness and criminal behaviour and special arrangements may be needed for the payment of rent arrears and compensation for damage. The housing and health departments of the local authority will give what support they can while in other cases the family may be taken under the wing of a voluntary organization such as a housing trust.

Safety in the Home

Many accidents which occur in the home, particularly to the very young and the elderly, could be prevented if sufficient precautions were taken. Mention has already been made of the importance of fixed guards round all fires where there are children (see p. 43). Windows should be guarded so that an active toddler cannot fall out. The risk of accidents is increased where there are steep stairs, faulty floors and poor lighting.

Housing for Special Groups

Many elderly people dislike leaving a home they may have lived in for many years even though it is too large for their needs and they can no longer manage the upkeep. Some local authorities have converted large houses into flatlets which are suitable for those living alone, while in other areas there are hostels which have communal dining- and sitting-rooms and individual centrally heated bedsitting-rooms. Perhaps the ideal accommodation for independent elderly people is a purpose-built group of individual units centred round a garden and with one flat or bungalow reserved for a warden. The houses should be centrally heated and have a built-in handrail for support when getting in and out of the bath. The windows should be low enough so that the occupant can see out when sitting down and the accommodation should be situated where the residents can see the world go by and not feel shut away from the rest of the community.

Disabled people need special housing arrangements according to their disability. Sliding doors which open to a width of at least one metre are needed where a wheelchair is in use and there must also be ramps instead of steps and sufficient width in the passage to turn the chair. The bathroom must be wide enough to allow the chair alongside and the lavatory should be in the same room, while the basin must allow the chair to slide underneath without catching. Cupboards must be of a suitable height to allow easy access for someone sitting in a wheelchair and there are a wide variety of gadgets available to help the disabled housewife. Central heating is important as immobile people may feel the cold. Carpets and rugs should be avoided and the floors can be treated to prevent the surface being slippery.

Ventilation

Efficient ventilation is necessary for comfortable living and working conditions and this means that there must be a regular interchange of air. The temperature and movement of the air as well as the amount of moisture it contains all affect the balance between heat lost and heat gained from the body. The cooler the air the greater the heat lost from the body; similarly cold walls absorb room heat and cool the room and warm walls help to maintain room temperature. Moving air helps the cooling process because it increases evaporation from the body surface. Air which is dry can absorb more water vapour so evaporation is more effective and cooling power increased. Moist air causes a reduction in cooling power. The discomfort which is felt in stuffy rooms is due to heat stagnation which is brought about by increased air temperature, excess moisture and lack of air movement all resulting in inadequate heat loss. Convection is the movement of air – or liquid – due to heating. Once heated, air becomes lighter and rises, cooler air taking its place and in turn becoming heated and rising (see Fig. 32). Radiation is the direct passage of heat from a warm object through the air to an object or person, which in turn becomes warm.

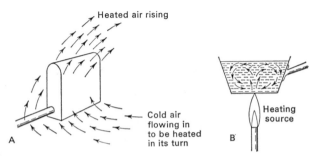

Heated air rising

Cold air flowing in to be heated in its turn

Heating source

A

B

32. Transmission of heat by convection; A, Air heating; B, Fluid heating.

When the atmospheric temperature is between 13 to 24°C (58° to 74°F) the greatest part of heat loss is by radiation; at higher temperatures heat loss by evaporation increases while at temperatures above 37°C (100°F) evaporation is the only method of losing heat. This explains why humidity is so important a factor, for a low humidity will assist evaporation and cooling but a high humidity will diminish heat loss. An atmospheric temperature of 29°C (82°F) in a high humidity is more uncomfortable than 43°C (110°F) in a low humidity.

Natural ventilation is aided by the provision of adequate air inlets and outlets. The inlet should be large enough to allow air to diffuse slowly but steadily throughout the room so that it does not cause a noticeable current of air, a draught. Windows and doors act as air inlets even when they are shut and will cause a draught if both are open opposite each other. Air is drawn out of a room through chimneys and ventilators, (see Fig. 33). Hot air rises and is replaced by colder, heavier air which makes a continual convection current around the room.

Air conditioning is an artificial method of ventilating a room or building. The temperature and moisture content of the air is regulated to a predetermined level and the air is then driven into the rooms by fans which blow it along air ducts. This

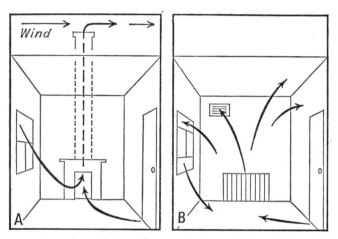

33. A, Natural ventilation of a room by convection currents up the chimney; B, Ventilation with central heating giving slower moving air.

system is often used in conjunction with the forcible extraction of air, particularly in places where large numbers of people gather such as cinemas, dance halls, and conference rooms.

Heating

Whatever method of heating is used in the home it should be possible to warm every room to 65° to 75°F (18° to 23°C). The type of heating used will depend on a variety of factors such as whether the heating is to be continuous or intermittent, the size of the room and whether the area has been designated a 'smokeless zone' or not (see Chapter 11).

Heat spreads from the source by radiation, convection and to a lesser extent by conduction. Convection is the most effective method, particularly if there is central heating, which is efficient and gives equal heat all over the house. It also warms the structure and reduces condensation and can be adjusted as the weather changes. It is, however, expensive to install and to run. Open coal fires are disappearing as smokeless zones increase, although smokeless fuel is available and some types of open fire will burn continuously and heat the water. This is not an efficient way of warming a house as much of the heat goes up the chimney. More and more use is being made of labour saving heaters such as gas and electric fires, night storage heaters and full central heating fired by oil, gas or electricity (see Fig. 34) Newer methods include under-floor heating and hot air ducts. It is economical to lag the roofspace with fibre-glass, though care must be taken if the water tank is in the roof, as cutting off the heat from the house may mean that the tank will freeze in winter. Double glazing also helps to keep houses warm as it reduces heat loss through windows; this can be quite substantial.

Lighting

Electricity is the only effective means of artificial lighting and it is particularly important for the elderly whose vision may be less good. Full use should be made of sunlight and all lighting is enhanced by light-coloured walls and surfaces which will reflect the light. A fluorescent light is valuable in kitchens and any place where food is handled as it gives a steady light with a minimum shadow. Wherever artificial light is used it

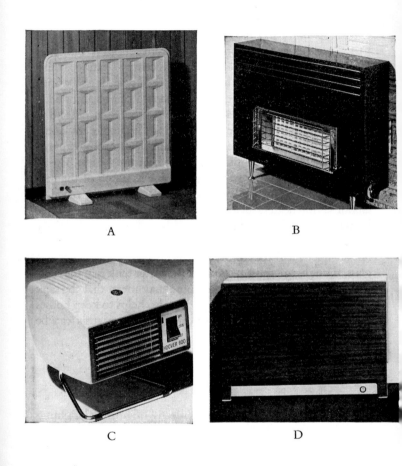

A

B

C

D

34. A selection of modern heating appliances; A, An oil–filled electric radiator; B, Gas convector heater; C, Electric fan heater; D, Electric storage heater.

must be sufficiently bright and without glare and there should be no flickering or shadow. For reading and any close work the light should shine over the left shoulder for right-handed people (see Fig. 35).

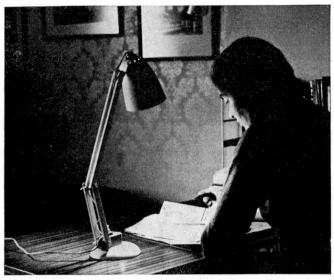

35. Adequate lighting for reading is required (T. Poyser).

Adequate lighting is important in factories and in the prevention of accidents.

11

The Environment

It was in the nineteenth century that it was first recognized that some of the most important measures which could be taken to improve the environment were efficient drainage, the removal of refuse and the provision of a pure water supply.

Water

The importance of a clean water supply was demonstrated conclusively during the cholera epidemic of 1844 when it was proved that water contaminated with faeces was the main cause of the spread of the disease. At the same time it was also shown that typhoid fever, which was a more common disease, was spread in the same way. Efforts were then made to improve both water supplies and the methods used for disposal of sewage.

If a pure water supply can be provided it almost ensures that diseases will not be spread in this way, but it is still a common method of spread in more primitive communities. The last serious waterborne outbreak of typhoid fever in Britain was in 1937 when 290 cases occurred in and around Croydon in Surrey. The carrier of the disease was a man working on a deep well which formed part of the town's water supply. In 1963 a waterborne outbreak in Zermatt, Switzerland resulted in 434 cases. Holidaymakers and people who travel in the remote areas of Spain, North Africa and the Middle and Far East are liable to typhoid and they should take the precaution of sterilizing water with appropriate chemicals and of receiving TAB vaccine before they leave for the journey. It is a recommendation of the Department of Health and Social Security that travellers to any part of Europe as well as to other more remote parts of the world should receive the vaccine before they travel.

Water Supplies

The provision of sufficient quantities of water inside every home is one of the most difficult environmental targets in the world. Where there is plenty of rain and modern methods of water storage and transportation there is usually sufficient water for every town and village, but where there is a dry climate with little rain, water is a precious commodity and it is often impure and unsafe.

Water is evaporated by the energy of the sun from the surfaces of the sea, lakes, rivers and moist ground and is precipitated as rain, hail, snow or dew. During these processes a certain amount of purification takes place. Some then returns to the atmosphere through further evaporation, some sinks into the soil and becomes underground water, some flows over the surface in the form of rivers and streams which may flow into lakes and remain as upland surface water, or flow on until it is eventually discharged back into the sea (see Fig. 36).

Underground water is that water which, having fallen as rain, sinks into the soil until it reaches an impermeable layer of rock, where it then forms an underground lake. In rural areas where there is no main water supply a shallow well may be sunk to tap this source of water but it may prove an unreliable source because if there is a prolonged drought the supply may dry up and there is always the possibility that the water in a shallow well may be contaminated by sewage. The terms shallow and deep do not refer to the actual depth of the well

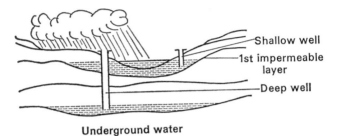

Underground water

36. Distribution of water underground.

but to the number of impermeable layers of rock through which the well shaft passes before it reaches the trapped water. A shallow well taps water trapped on the first impermeable layer, a deep well taps water lying below the first impermeable layer and an artesian well taps water from below the second impermeable layer which is under pressure. Some purification of well water occurs as the water passes through the soil, so the deeper the well the more pure the water is likely to be, but well water also tends to be hard because of the quantity of dissolved mineral substances it contains.

River water is used to supply many towns and about two-thirds of London's water comes from the Thames or its tributaries. River water, however, is usually polluted with sewage, dirt from the towns through which it has passed and industrial waste and it is frequently hard, containing many dissolved minerals.

Upland surface water is found in hilly areas where the rainwater running off the surface is collected in lakes which may be natural or manmade. Most artificial lakes are found in uninhabited mountainous areas and are dependent on the construction of a dam across the mouth of a valley. The land lying behind the dam becomes flooded and the water can then be piped to wherever it is needed. Liverpool and Birmingham both get water in this way from lakes in North Wales.

During the process of collection the quality of the water may be altered. Rainwater collects dirt, bacteria and gases in solution from the atmosphere through which it passes. Near towns it picks up soot and smoke and other mineral and organic matter is collected from the land over which it flows. Near the sea salts are absorbed from sea spray. Mention has already been made of the possibility of water supplies being contaminated with sewage and of the danger of certain diseases being spread in this way; the absorption of mineral salts which make the water hard has also been mentioned. Hard water creates problems because the salts may be precipitated when the water is boiled and this causes the 'furring' of kettles, water pipes and boilers and also excessive amounts of soap are required to produce a lather in hard water. The addition of lime to the water precipitates the calcium and magnesium and makes the water softer.

Water Requirements

The minimum amount of water required to maintain life is about two litres (3 to 4 pints) per person per day. Under normal circumstances vast quantities of water are used for purposes other than drinking, such as cooking, washing, laundry, flushing lavatories, washing up and cleaning the house and car. The use of washing machines and garden hoses increases this domestic quantity. Water is also used for street cleaning and fire fighting and swimming pools; industrial concerns use large amounts, often having an individual supply from a river or a well. When this water has been used it is returned to rivers or the sea as sewage effluent or industrial waste and occasionally this wastewater may pass into the ground. Serious health risks may result from the extraction of water from rivers or wells which have been contaminated in this way.

Water Purification

Between the collection of water and its distribution to the user, water must be purified so that it is safe. Following collection from a river water is first strained by passing it through various types of screens to entrap fish, twigs and other floating objects. Storage of the water provides the reserve necessary for a constant supply and also helps in the purification process because the impurities and suspended matter sink to the bottom and the wind and sunshine prohibit the growth of bacteria. When it is to be used the water is filtered through tanks containing sand which has on its surface a layer of jelly-like organic matter which holds up the impurities. Periodically this layer is scraped off and the sand is washed, but the layer must form again before the sand filter will be effective. Sand filters are being replaced by chemical filters which set more quickly. A chemical substance such as aluminium silicate forms the jelly-like layer and this type of filter can be cleaned by passing compressed air through the filter in the reverse direction. Disinfection is carried out by adding a measured dose of chlorine to the water, which oxidizes the organic matter and kills pathogenic bacteria, although it is not effective against amoebic cysts and some viruses. The chlorine is introduced at least one hour before the water is withdrawn to give it time to act. Other methods of disinfection less commonly used include the use of ozone and ultraviolet rays, while boiling will sterilize the water in an emergency. Regular sampling of the water is carried out to test it for bacterial and chemical purity.

Fluoridation

The amount of fluoride found naturally in the water affects the incidence of dental caries. In areas where the fluoride content is high the amount of dental caries is considerably reduced. In areas where the content is low some authorities have added the substance to water supplies to bring the concentration up to one part per million. There have been complaints about this on the grounds that it is an intrusion into individual liberty.

Water which is lacking in iodine may be a danger to health as the thyroid gland needs this substance to function normally. This is most likely to occur in areas which are some distance from the sea, notably Derbyshire in Britain, and Switzerland in Europe, and the difficulty may be overcome by adding iodine to table salt.

Water distribution

When the water is ready for use it is carried from the treatment plant to a service reservoir which is situated on high ground, or it may be stored in a water tower. This ensures that there is an adequate pressure in the mains and forms a reserve for fire fighting as well as making sure that there will not be any interruption in the supply. Water is distributed from the service reservoir in large water mains which are carefully laid and sealed so that there is no danger of contamination from sewers, which frequently run beside the mains under the road. From the mains a service pipe carries water into the storage cistern in each house and there is usually a stopcock at the boundary of the property so that the water can be turned off if necessary. The domestic storage cistern is usually in the roof space, which helps to maintain an even pressure in the pipes and fixtures throughout the house, but there is usually one tap in the kitchen which is supplied directly from the mains.

Sewage

Where water is freely available the water carriage system is the most effective way of transferring sewage from domestic premises. In a combined system wastewater from sinks, lavatories and baths is combined with rainwater from streets and roofs and is carried into a main sewer where it flows towards the treatment works. These works are usually on the outskirts of towns and near streams or rivers and the end product of sewage treatment should be a clean safe liquid which can be passed into the stream without harm.

The pipes carrying wastewater from all parts of the house pour their contents into the house drain which in turn empties into the main sewer. Where the house pipes meet the house drain and again where the house drain meets the sewer, there is an inspection chamber with a removable metal cover to enable the drains to be cleaned. About 30 to 50 gallons of wastewater and sewage per person per day is poured into the sewage system, this amount increases considerably when there is a rainstorm. The sewers are laid to follow the downward slope of the land so that gravity flow aided by pumping conveys the water to the treatment plant. There are manholes every 100 yards or so to allow inspection and cleaning of the sewer.

Sewage Treatment

The raw sewage is first passed through a screening process during which coarse particles and larger solids are removed. In some cases these may be shredded and returned to the flow to be dealt with at a later stage. In a combined sewerage system grit from the roads may be a problem, causing heavy wear in pumps; to get rid of it the sewage is passed slowly along a narrow channel which allows the grit to settle but the lighter solids to flow on in the water. The sewage then flows into large tanks where the solid matter (sludge) is separated from the liquid matter (effluent). The remaining water is extracted from the sludge and the dried material may be treated and used as fertilizer or it may be dumped at sea. The effluent is purified by filtration through tanks containing stones and chippings in graduated sizes, during which time the natural cleansing processes of bacterial action and oxidation render the liquid safe to be discharged into rivers or streams.

In some seaside areas treated sewage is discharged into the sea. This is done well below the low water line and only at ebb tide, but even with these precautions there is some danger of pollution of the beaches. Constant chemical and bacterial sampling is carried out to ensure that the sewage is safe for disposal.

In rural areas where there is no main drainage system the sewage is carried in pipes from the house to a watertight storage tank called a cesspool where anaerobic bacteria act on the organic material. The cesspool must be emptied regularly by pumping the contents into a sewage tanker which then takes the sewage to the treatment works for disposal. A septic tank is similar to a cesspool but does not need to be emptied.

After treatment by anaerobic bacteria the contents are deemed safe and are allowed to drain away into adjoining ground. Chemical closets are useful for those who live in caravans or houseboats or who enjoy camping. Caustic soda or coal tar is used to disinfect the contents and liquefy the solid matter.

Refuse

In recent years the collection of refuse has become an increasing problem because of the greater use of disposable items and packaging materials and the decrease in the number of houses which have facilities for burning rubbish (Fig. 37).

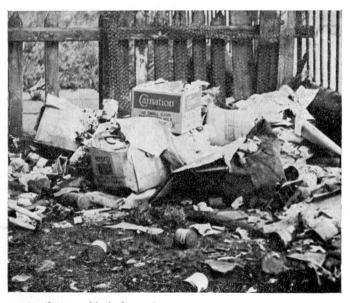

37. Inefficient rubbish disposal.

Rubbish bins for domestic use must be sound and have well-fitting lids to keep out vermin, flies and cats. Some local authorities supply strong paper bags in a metal frame with a lid, which reduces the handling as the bag can be removed and a new one put in its place. It may also be necessary to protect the bag with a wire mesh frame to prevent animals gnawing through the paper to get at the contents. In other areas polythene sacks are provided to line the bins so that again the whole sack can be exchanged for a new one. The rubbish is collected in specially designed vehicles to reduce the dust and scattering of rubbish and so that they can be emptied easily when they reach the disposal works. Many of these vans contain mechanism for grinding the contents down immediately so that more can be carried in one van.

Refuse Disposal

This is carried out in a variety of ways. The metal objects may be separated out with the help of an electromagnet and sold for scrap. The remaining material may be incinerated at a very high temperature until only clinker remains which may then be used in roadbuilding.

An alternative method of disposal is by controlled tipping in which the refuse is deposited in a layer not more than six feet thick, this is then sealed on all sides with at least nine inches of earth. The refuse must be covered as quickly as possible, always within 72 hours, to prevent danger from fire or infestation with vermin or flies. This method may be used to level uneven land or to fill quarries.

Refuse may also be disposed of by dumping at sea but this must be far enough out to prevent contaminating beaches.

Air

In many cities and industrial areas air is so dirty and contains so many impurities that it can endanger health. Industrial haze is created by smoke and fumes from vehicle exhaust pipes and from household and factory chimneys. City air contains soot, lead, sulphur and carbon monoxide among other substances and there is more chronic bronchitis among town dwellers than among country dwellers.

Weather affects atmospheric pollution because the impurities become trapped underneath fog and their concentration builds up. Those people who are healthy may be little affected by these conditions but for those who suffer from chronic bronchitis and whose condition is always worse in the damp fogs of winter, the additional inhalation of smoke particles irritates the bronchial mucosa even further. In December 1952 there was a period of 'smog' which lasted five days and during that time 4000 people died in the London area alone as a direct result of the smog. Atmospheric pollution also plays a small but definite part in the production of lung cancer.

Control of Pollution

Efforts to reduce air pollution have been made in many areas with noticeable effects. Coal-burning steam engines have been replaced by electric and diesel locomotives. The creation of smokeless zones under the 'Clean Air Act' has made a valuable contribution to the improvement of the air we breathe. Before any area can be designated as a 'smoke control area' adequate quantities of suitable alternative fuel must be ensured. Up to 70 per cent of the cost of alterations is paid to a householder who has to change the method of heating in his house. Old fire grates must be replaced with ones capable of

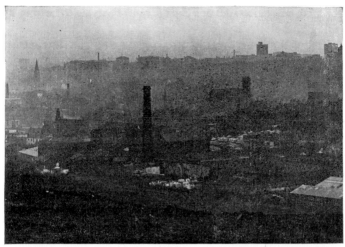

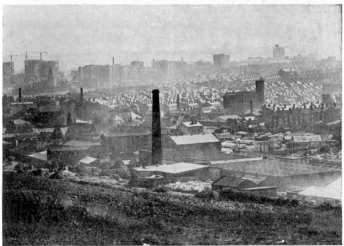

38. Two views of the same landscape in Leeds contrasting the atmospheric conditions before and after implementation of the Clean Air Act.

burning smokeless fuel or a change must be made to heating by oil, gas or electricity.

Regulations affecting industrial premises restrict the emission of dark smoke to a maximum of ten minutes in any eight-hour period and never for more than four minutes continuously. Prior approval must be given for the installation of furnaces and boilers unless they can be operated without making smoke. The local authority may also specify the height of any industrial chimney being built so that gases are carried away from centres of population.

Those towns where smoke control areas have been established show a marked improvement in atmospheric pollution (Fig. 38), but the programme is slow because of the shortage of smokeless fuels, the general energy crisis and stringent financial limitations.

12

Food Hygiene

Food hygiene is usually taken to mean those aspects of food production and handling which deal with the prevention of foodborne infections and diseases caused by chemical poisons, but food affects health in more ways than that (see also Chapter 5). An important aspect of food hygiene is cultural in origin. Foods that are safe and wholesome may not be aesthetically acceptable to people of other races and tradition and religious beliefs play a considerable part in food standards and sanitation practices. The main objective is to ensure the production and distribution of safe, clean and wholesome food and to this end it is necessary to prevent contamination and to ensure that microorganisms which exist in or contaminate food in spite of all precautions are not allowed to increase to a level which will cause ill effects.

The producer, the processor, the manufacturer, the transport agencies and the retailer are all involved and education of these people is the most important single factor. Legislation has a big part to play but laws alone will not be enough unless people understand and believe in the reasons behind the legislation and are willing to play their part.

Food production

Milk is a valuable food because the carbohydrate, protein and fat are in balanced and easily assimilated proportions and because it is rich in calcium and phosphorus. Because of the way in which it is produced and because of its food value milk is a good medium for the growth of bacteria and it therefore presents a special problem.

By law cow's milk must contain not less than 3 per cent butterfat and no colouring matter, water or preservative may be added. Dairy farmers must be registered and milk production must be up to a certain standard. In order to attain this the cows must be free from disease and must be reared in a clean environment. Tuberculosis has virtually disappeared from herds in Britain and brucellosis, which is now rather more common, can be prevented from infecting humans by pasteurization of milk. The cleanliness of the cows, the equipment and the workers during milking is all checked regularly. The milk must be cooled promptly after milking and is kept cool until it is collected and taken to the local centre for treatment.

Local authorities register milk distributors and have certain responsibilities if milk is infected, or suspected of being infected, with disease. A dairy worker must notify the local authority if he contracts food poisoning, gastroenteritis and other specified diseases. Any employee may be medically examined if he is suspected of suffering from a disease likely to cause infection in milk. If anyone is found to be suffering from a disease caused by milk consumption that milk may be prohibited from being used for human consumption.

Milk may be treated in a variety of ways to render it free from infection.

Pasteurization is the most common method. The milk is kept at a temperature of not less than 71·5°C (161°F) for at least 15 seconds and is then immediately cooled to at least 10°C (50°F). It is then put into sterilized containers which are sealed and stored in a cool place until they are delivered. This method is known as the High Temperature Short Time Method (HTST). An alternative way is to raise the temperature of the milk to 62·8° to 65·5°C (145° to 150°F) for 30 minutes and then to cool it rapidly to not more than 10°C (50°F). This is called the Holder Method. Pasteurization destroys all pathogenic bacteria including *Mycobacterium tuberculosis, Brucella abortus, streptococci, staphylococci, Salmonella typhi* and *S. paratyphi* and *Corynebacterium diphtheriae,* but the taste and appearance remain unaltered.

Sterilization of milk involves heating it to 108·9°C (228°F) for 10 to 12 minutes before it is cooled. The milk is first homogenized so that the fat is distributed uniformly throughout, and is bottled and sealed so that if the bottles remain unopened the milk will keep for a long period, but this method does affect the flavour and colour of the milk to some extent.

A more recent development is the **ultra-heat treatment** in which the milk is kept at 132°C (270°F) for not less than 1 second and is then placed in sterile containers in which it is sold to the public.

Untreated milk can still be bought in containers which are labelled 'farm bottled'. The milk is bottled, immediately after milking and cooling, into unventilated containers in which it will be sold.

Other milk products such as ice-cream are also subject to strict regulations. It must not contain less than 5 per cent fat and must be pasteurized before being frozen. Butter must contain no more than 16 per cent moisture and no preservatives or colouring matter.

All **meat** is examined before it is sold and notice must be given when animals are to be slaughtered in order to facilitate inspection. Slaughter houses are licensed and inspected regularly. All imported meat must bear the officially recognized certificate of the country of origin and this must show that the meat was inspected before and after slaughter and that necessary precautions were taken in the preparation and packing of the meat to prevent endangering the health of the public. Prompt and efficient refrigeration plays an important part in this process. Food control agencies are also concerned about such changing problems as the use of hormones and antibiotics in feeding animals and poultry and the residues of poisonous chemicals on fruit and vegetables which have been treated with pesticides.

Eggs must be sold while they are still fresh or if imported in liquid form the product must be pasteurized.

Margarine is made of animal and vegetable fats to which milk has been added and it must not contain more than 10 per cent water or 10 per cent butter fat. It is usually fortified with vitamins A and D.

Substances such as **shellfish** may be infected with Salmonela if they have been collected from areas which are contaminated with sewage. An order prevents the collection of shellfish from such areas.

Random sampling of food, drink and drugs is carried out by public health inspectors and chemical analysis and bacteriological tests check legal requirements. Adulteration of food is not common and when it does occur is usually accidental. The addition of preservatives and colouring matter is subject to strict control and only limited amounts may be used in certain specified foods.

Food Personnel Handling

The most important factors in the production and distribution of clean food are the people who handle the food during all the stages from source to consumer. Each person in this chain must be scrupulously clean with particular attention paid to the hands and fingernails. The clothes which are worn for work must be clean and the hair clean and covered with a

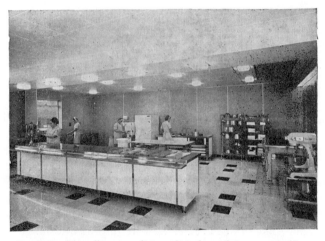

39. Good food handling conditions (Marks and Spencer Ltd.).

clean cap or tied up in a clean scarf. There must be no smoking where food is handled or where it is lying on open shelves or trays. No handkerchiefs should be allowed in kitchens but paper ones should be used and disposed of immediately, before washing the hands. Food should be handled as little as possible and tongs or forks should be used whenever possible. A clean, efficient kitchen for food preparation is shown in Fig. 39.

Any wound or cut must be completely sealed by a water-proof dressing to enable the hands to be washed freely. It is important that such personnel understand the ways in which food can become contaminated and they are taught the importance of their own role in preventing such contamination. They must be convinced of the importance of clean personal habits and of reporting any illness such as sore throats, colds and gastroenteritis. If food is contaminated in the kitchen of a private house it is only the immediate family who will be affected; if the food in a factory, restaurant or shop is contaminated thousands may be affected.

In order for the personnel to maintain high standards of personal hygiene the facilities within the building must be adequate. There must be an ample supply of hot water conveniently situated and the lavatories and washbasins must be properly constructed and maintained in a clean condition. Soap and towels must be freely available and proper lighting and ventilation are also necessary. The lavatories must not be in direct communication with the food rooms. A supply of suitable waterproof dressings for small wounds must be available.

The premises in which food is handled must be soundly constructed and free of vermin. All food and beverage establishments including street vendors, vans and food vending machines have to be licensed and are inspected to make sure they are up to the required standard. Ventilation must be ample and in many cases will need to be assisted by mechanical means such as extractor fans. Lighting must be adequate; fluorescent light is usually the most suitable. The walls and floors of food rooms must be kept clean and are best made of an easily washable, impermeable material. The equipment must be in good repair so that it can be kept clean and the most effective way of washing equipment is by the use of a mechanical washer which renders the items virtually sterile when the cycle is complete. Adequate shelving and other storage space, preferably enclosed and dustproof, must be available as it is against the regulations for food to be placed lower than eighteen inches from the floor. Unpackaged food which is sold must be wrapped in clean paper and must not be in contact with newsprint, unless it is uncooked vegetables.

Preservation of food

There are a variety of methods for preserving food.

Freezing or **chilling** is an effective and convenient method as the bacteria cannot multiply at low temperatures. Frozen food is brought to a temperature of minus 4·4°C (24°F) or below and the taste of the food is not altered if freezing is carried out quickly. A quick freezing process is carried out for retail packs and it is very popular. Freezing takes place at very low temperatures so that the food passes through the critical phase of 0° to —5°C (32° to 23°F) within 1½ to 2 hours. Once frozen food is thawed bacterial multiplication starts again so the food must be cooked and eaten as soon as it is thawed. Food which is partially cooked and then kept warm is one of the most likely sources of bacterial contamination. The conditions of warmth, humidity and nourishment are just those which bacteria need to increase in number to a point which may cause harm to the individual who eats the food. Once cooked, food should be eaten immediately or cooled quickly and stored in a refrigerator until required. Chilled food is brought to a temperature of —3° to —1°C (28° to 30°F).

High temperatures are used in canning processes. The food is put into the cans and then cooked, sterilized and sealed. The food will remain sound if the can is properly sealed and air cannot enter. The cans are often cooled under water and it is important that the water must be pure. An outbreak of typhoid in Aberdeen was traced to a tin of corned beef and was probably caused by the entry of unclean water into the tin through a small pinhole as the cans were cooled in river water before import.

Some food is preserved by **curing** or **smoking** which enhances the flavour and inhibits the growth of micro-organisms. Bacon, ham and fish are commonly treated in this way.

Drying is an effective way of preserving substances such as egg, milk, meat, fish, fruit and vegetables. Bacterial growth is inhibited by the lack of moisture and this method does not appreciably alter the vitamin content.

Air conditioning is used to enable certain types of fruit and vegetables to be maintained in good condition and this method has also been applied to milk.

Irradiation is a method which is being developed for preservation of some foods and for the elimination of vermin and the prevention of spoilage.

13

Health and Social Services

National Health Service

The National Health Service is probably the most renowned of Britain's social services. It provides comprehensive health care, in both hospital and community for everyone, irrespective of social status and without regard to any insurance payment.

The development of a national health service followed the Second World War because the inadequacy of existing services had become apparent. Hospitals were lacking in both staff and resources and community health services varied widely from district to district. The need for complete reshaping of medical and health services was accepted and the general pattern for reorganization was set out in a report by William Beveridge (1942). A final health service plan was evolved by Aneurin Bevan and the National Health Service Act was passed in 1946. The service came into being in 1948 and was based on a tripartite system of administration, corresponding to the three main parts of the service. The responsibility for hospitals rested with Regional Hospital Boards and Hospital Management Committees and with Boards of Governors for Teaching Hospitals. Executive

Councils were responsible for the general medical services provided by general practitioners, dentists and pharmacists. and county councils and county boroughs for the local authority health services. All three sections of the service were responsible to the Minister of Health in the central government department.

For 25 years following its inception the administration of the National Health Service remained virtually unchanged but during this time one of the main problems proved to be the basic tripartite nature of the service. Each section of the service operated through its own administrative body and lack of liaison between the three frequently produced problems which related directly to patient care. For example, until 1959 it was difficult for general practitioners to have access to the medical notes of patients admitted to psychiatric hospitals but it is the general practitioner who has the job of maintaining the patient's health in the community following discharge, a difficult task without full and accurate knowledge of the cause of the illness and its treatment. Similarly family doctors and community nurses are frequently able to offer their hospital colleagues valuable information concerning a patient's social circumstances which may aid diagnosis and subsequent treatment. Thus each section of the service has its own contribution to make towards the total welfare of the patient. In recent years the importance of crossing the administrative barriers that exist between hospital and community medicine has been realized and from April 1974 a reorganized, unified National Health Service has been operating.

Unification of the National Health Service

The unification of National Health Service administration draws together within a single structure the administration of family practitioner services, local authority services, hospital services and the school health service. Former administrative bodies, i.e. Regional Hospital Boards, Hospital Management Committees and Boards of Governors were phased out and replaced by Regional and Area Health Authorities, responsible for administering all three branches of the service. Executive councils also disappeared and were replaced by Family Practitioner Committees who will be responsible to the Area Health Authorities.

The Department of Health and Social Security continues as the central government department responsible for overall planning. The Secretary of State for the Department determines health policy and is responsible to Parliament for the Health Service. He is responsible, among other things, for the provision of adequate accommodation for any service under the National Health Service, for medical, dental, nursing and ambulance services, for facilities for the care of expectant and nursing mothers and their babies and for the prevention of illness and the after-care of people who have been ill. School health services and family planning services also come under his jurisdiction.

Expert committees are set up as necessary to advise on special problems. One such committee is the Central Health Services Council which consists of professional people from all major medical, nursing, dental and pharmaceutical organizations and others with special experience in hospital management or community health services. This council advises the Secretary of State on all important matters concerning the National Health Service and makes an annual report.

There are also several standing advisory committees each dealing with specialist topics such as child health, maternity and midwifery services and mental health. Special *ad hoc* committees may also be appointed, as the need arises, to study special subjects and to make recommendations.

The basic unit in the unified health service is the District, a

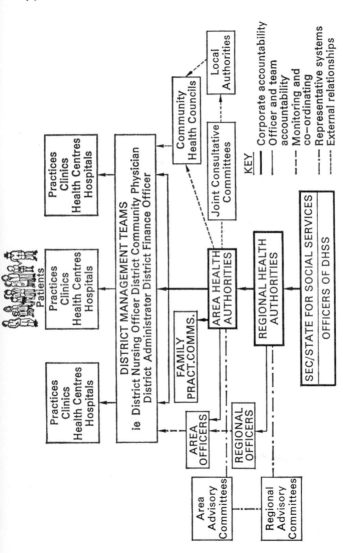

40. Framework of NHS structure following reorganization (Department of Management Studies, North London Polytechnic).

term which describes the geographical area served by one District General Hospital. Each district is controlled by a District Management Team (DMT) of officers who are responsible for the day to day management of hospital and community services. Each DMT is composed of six officers; one consultant and one family practitioner, a District Nursing Officer, a District Community Physician, a District Administrator and a District Treasurer. It is responsible for the services and no one member is the managerial superior of another.

The number of Districts which form one Area varies but in most cases is more than one. Where there is only one District General Hospital in an Area the management of the services in that Area is the responsibility of the Area Team of Officers and there is no District Management Team.

There are 90 Area Health Authorities (AHA) in England and they are responsible for all hospital services and all community health services. Some are designated Area Health Authority (Teaching) and are centres for medical teaching in conjunction with the corresponding university.

In most cases the AHA corresponds to the area of a new local authority which is responsible for social services and education. The exceptions to this are in London, where there are 32 London boroughs but only 16 AHAs, and on Merseyside.

The chairman of each AHA is appointed by the Secretary of State after consultation with the chairman of the Regional Health Authority. There are about 15 members, four appointed by the local authority and the university where there is one. The rest are appointed by the Regional Health Authority after consultation with health professions and other organizations.

Each AHA is serviced by an Area Team of Officers (ATO), an Area Medical Officer, Area Nursing Officer, Area Administrator and Area Treasurer. This team is the planning and evaluation team for the AHA and will draw up planning guide lines for each District. However the DMT are directly responsible to the AHAs and not to the ATO which advises the AHA independently.

England is divided into 14 Regions each having a Regional Health Authority (RHA) which is responsible for the allocation of money to its constituent AHAs, for capital building programmes and for postgraduate training of medical, dental and nursing staff. The Chairman and members of each RHA are appointed by the Secretary of State after consultation with local authorities, universities and the main health professions.

The Regional Team of Officers (RTO) is formed of five people; the Regional Medical Officer, the Regional Nursing Officer, the Works Officer, the Administrator and the Treasurer. They are responsible for preparing regional development plans and for monitoring the programmes of the AHAs.

In Wales there is no RHA but there are 8 AHAs. Scotland has 14 simple Health Boards.

Communications

Recent reforms in health and social services have served to emphasize the need for close liaison between all branches of the service. Nurses have a particular role to play as direct providers of care but that role is only one link in the chain that leads from the sick patient to the healthy individual restored to active life in the community.

Nursing staff in hospital must realize the importance of contacting and giving adequate information to community colleagues before a patient is discharged so that continuity of care is assured. Similarly the community health team should feel able to approach hospital staff for specific help and advice.

It is important also for nurses to know the source of rehabilitative services and to check that any community service required has been arranged before discharge.

The advent of the 'district general hospital' in the new structure should promote hospital–community relations and the recent attachment of district nurses and health visitors to specialized units has ensured follow-up care.

Social Services

The Local Authority Social Service Act was passed in 1970 following the report of a committee set up under the chairmanship of Frederick Seebohm to examine the organization and workings of the personal social services. The Committee reported that the development of the social services during the postwar years had been that of isolated response to a particular need and that the resulting service was fragmented and divided between the different departments of health, welfare, nursing and education. In practice this meant that a family with multiple problems might be receiving help from several different caseworkers, a situation which could lead to confusion and failure to give support to the family as a whole. The report of the Seebohm Committee therefore recommended the setting up of a single new department, to be called the Department of Social Services which would aim to provide a wide variety of help to persons or families in need. The report also stressed that social casework should be geared to helping families, rather than concentrating on one particular problem which may represent only one isolated facet of a family's total need.

The new departments, which came into being in 1971, took over the work of the children's department and services for the elderly and homeless, work previously carried out by local authority health departments, i.e. the home help service, mental health social work, provision of day nurseries, supervision of child minders, meals-on-wheels and laundry service. Residential care of all types is also provided by the new departments.

Following the passing of the Chronic Sick and Disabled Persons Act, 1971, local authority social services departments have a duty to discover the number of disabled people in their areas and to provide resources to meet their needs. Social service departments are therefore responsible for providing special equipment, telephones, aids and adaptations in the home, television, libraries and recreational facilities. Workshops and residential accommodation must be made available and new local authority buildings such as cinemas and theatres must be adapted to meet the needs of the disabled.

The local authority employs teams of social workers to run these services, who work from an area social services office. An area office should be easily accessible and should serve a population of between 50 000 and 100 000 people, with a team of at least 10 to 12 social workers.

Social services departments should also make use of local voluntary organizations. The role of voluntary bodies is an important one since they provide valuable support to local authority services in certain specific areas of need. The Family Service Unit and the Family Welfare Association give intensive support to small groups of families with multiple problems. The National Society for the Prevention of Cruelty to Children may be called in to give help when the problem is one of child deprivation or neglect. Various other specific organizations give financial aid and support when appropriate, e.g. Invalid Children's Aid Association, British Diabetic Association and the Association for Spina Bifida and Hydrocephalus.

National Insurance

The provision of a national insurance scheme has an indirect effect on the health of the nation by removing the fear of complete loss of wages by reason of illness, injury or unemployment. The National Insurance Act of 1946, which took effect in 1948 at the same time as the National Health Service, provided for such a comprehensive system of insurance against loss of income by the inclusion of sickness and unemployment benefits, maternity benefits and retirement pensions. The insurance is compulsory and includes almost every one from school-leaving age to retirement.

Regular contribution throughout working life entitles anyone who is permanently resident in Britain to free treatment in a hospital within the National Health Service. General practitioners provide a service which is available to anyone. Most adult patients must pay part of the cost of any dental treatment which may be required, but children and expectant and nursing mothers do not pay.

Sight testing is free. There is a part charge for glasses which varies according to the type of lens needed and the frames chosen. Help with charges is given to those receiving supplementary pensions and family income supplements, and glasses are supplied free to children.

Prescription charges are payable at a standard rate for most adults, but are free for children, pensioners and certain other groups who are exempt from charges.

Items such as the provision of free milk for some children and inexpensive school dinners are mentioned in the appropriate chapters.

Health Team

In the new National Health Service community medical and nursing services are administered through the Regional and Area Health Authorities. Each area has an Area Medical Officer responsible for organizing the medical services, for advising the local authorities and for engaging in research programmes (as described earlier in the chapter). At Area and

District level a medical specialist in community medicine will be responsible for coordinating the preventive health services including vaccination and immunization, screening programmes, health education and chiropody. The general practitioner service is administered by the Area Health Authority through the Family Practitioner Committee and at Area and District levels nursing officers coordinate all aspects of the nursing services.

General Practitioner. The general practitioner is a qualified doctor responsible for providing domiciliary medical care to the patients on his list. Any person over the age of 16 is free to choose his own doctor and a list of general practitioners in a given locality is obtainable from the post office.

A general practitioner may work alone or in a group practice and there may be a health visitor, a midwife and a district nurse attached to the practice. Such a group constitutes the 'community health team'.

Midwife. The district midwife is a State Registered Nurse who has taken extra training of one year and having passed examinations set by the Central Midwives Board, may call herself a State Certified Midwife (SCM). She is responsible for the care of mothers and babies throughout pregnancy and childbirth and for 10 days afterwards; after this time care is handed over to the health visitor. The midwife meets expectant mothers at the antenatal clinic where she supervises antenatal care. She may also assist in the organization of classes in relaxation and mothercraft.

District Nurse. The district nurse may be either a State Registered or State Enrolled Nurse who has undertaken district nurse training in the area of her choice. The training lasts three months and leads to the National Certificate in

District Nursing. The district nurse tends the sick in their own homes, giving the basic nursing care such as blanket bathing, injections and dressings. She also has a subsidiary role as a health teacher since she can do much to educate her patients and their families during her visits. Patients are referred to the district nursing service by their general practitioners and the nurse works closely with him, reporting any significant changes in the patient's condition. She may also refer patients to the health visitor or to other social agencies.

In rural areas one person may combine the duties of district nurse/midwife.

The service is now administered by the Area Health Authority but until 1967 the training of district nurses was undertaken by the Queen's Institute of District Nursing. At the present time the Institute engages in research and offers refresher courses, and no longer trains home nurses.

Health Visitor. The health visitor holds a unique position in the health service being primarily concerned with the prevention of illness. She works alongside other members of the health team as a health educator and adviser both in the home and in the welfare clinic.

The health visitor's mutual contact with a family occurs most often after the birth of a baby, when she is notified by the hospital or district midwife. She then undertakes home visiting for the purpose of advising on child care and to acquaint the family with the services available to them at the local infant welfare clinic. As a result of this first contact she may be called upon to advise on many other problems of family life.

The health visitor is concerned with teaching the principles of healthy living to mothers, children and to the elderly. She offers support to families or individuals during periods of stress and undertakes follow-up visiting to those recently discharged from hospital and to the mentally sick. She is in a position 'to detect the early signs of ill health, abnormal development or social distress' and to refer to the appropriate agency for dealing with the problem. Similarly patients may be referred to her from general practitioners, hospital staff and social workers.

The health visitor may also undertake work in schools organizing discussion groups in topics such as mothercraft, smoking and sex education. The health visitor may work from a local clinic, her visiting being confined to several streets in the immediate vicinity, or she may be attached to a group of general practitioners in which case she visits only those patients on her doctor's list.

Health visitor training is undertaken at a university or college of technology and lasts one year. Candidates must be State Registered Nurses and hold either an obstetric certificate, Part 1 of midwifery training or be a State Certified Midwife.

Public Health Inspector. The work of the public health inspector is concerned with those services relating to environmental health, i.e. housing, water supply, food supply and infectious disease.

The public health inspector visits houses whenever there has been a complaint of insanitary conditions and then takes steps to compel the house owner to correct the deficiencies. He is concerned with the problems of overcrowding, the state of repair of property and any infestation by rats or mice.

The public health inspector is responsible for ensuring that every new house has an adequate water supply and he undertakes the inspection of sewage disposal works. He also visits shops, factories and restaurants where food is prepared or handled to ensure that this is done under hygienic conditions. In cases of infectious disease he may assist with the disinfection of infected premises.

The members of the health team, particularly those involved

in community nursing, have an unrivalled opportunity to see the patient in the context of his own environment and his family and to develop a deeper relationship between nurse and patient than is often possible in hospital. There is also the satisfaction of seeing a job through and the challenge and responsibility which accompanies the need to rely on one's own professional judgment and the greater flexibility of routine and of approach.

Statistics

The fact that diseases occur unequally throughout different social classes and different geographical areas shows that there are many social and climatic aspects of disease, many of which are imperfectly understood. The assessment of the health of a community can only be undertaken with the help of figures showing the births and deaths and the incidence of disease in that community.

The figures can be divided into three main groups. Those concerned with population, marriages and fertility are often known as **demographic** statistics. **Mortality** statistics are the figures relating to the numbers of deaths and the causes, while the incidence of disease, the number of people injured and incapacitated and the number admitted to hospital are included in the **morbidity** figures.

These figures can be obtained in a variety of ways. *Registration* of all births, deaths and marriages is compulsory in Britain. Birth registration is usually carried out by one or other parent who goes to the local Register office and registers the birth and receives a birth certificate for the child. *Notification* of the birth is also made by the doctor or midwife in attendance, to the local authority. Information about births is exchanged freely between the Registrar and the local authority and this enables visits to be made by the health visitor to advise on the care of the baby and the health of the mother. All deaths must also be *registered*. A relative is given a certificate showing the cause of death by the doctor and this certificate is taken to the local registrar, or may be sent by post, within five days. A death certificate is then issued which must be shown to the undertaker before burial or cremation can take place.

A complete set of statistics is obtained every ten years when the *census* is taken. The first census was taken in Britain in 1801 and has been repeated at ten year intervals ever since, with the exception of 1941 when the country was at war. Of the mass of figures obtained in this way the information of most value to those interested in public health is the numerical description of the population and its social, environmental and economic characteristics and the figures showing the mortality and morbidity rates from which the numbers of deaths or illnesses can be calculated in relation to the number of people at risk. A noticeable feature of population change in England and Wales in this century is the decreasing proportion of young people and the increasing proportion of the elderly. In 1881 out of every 100 people only 5 were over 65; in 1961, 12 out of every 100 were over 65.

A *sickness survey* shows the amount of ill health in a representative sample of people. One such survey went on continuously from 1944 to 1952, during which time a different sample of about 4000 adults was interviewed each month by field workers from the Central Office of Information. The information was obtained from the people themselves rather than from clinical records or medical notifications because one aim was to assess the amount of minor ill health which does not require medical care, in addition to that which does.

Other ways in which figures are obtained are through special returns. These include notification of infectious disease, certificates of incapacity for work, hospital admissions

and outpatient attendances. Since 1945 there has been a
national scheme for the registration of cancer patients who are
receiving treatment as hospital inpatients or outpatients. This
enables data to be collected on the incidence of cancer by site,
sex, age and stage of disease and to calculate survival rates.

In England and Wales the government department responsible for statistics is the General Register Office and the head of
the department is the Registrar General, who is a permanent
civil servant. Other countries have similar arrangements
though the titles may be different. International statistics are
compiled by an office of the United Nations Organization and
also by the World Health Organization and are published
annually. The world population which was about 2990
million in 1960, is estimated at about 5965 million by the year
2000. This doubling of the world population in less than half
a century will produce new problems in international public
health.

Birth Rates

The *birth rate* is derived from the registration of births and the
number given is the number of babies born alive for every
1000 people. It is calculated by dividing the number of live
births by the number of the population and multiplying by
1000.

$$\text{Live birth rate per 1000 population} = \frac{\text{No. of live births}}{\text{No. of population}} \times 1000$$

The figure was 28.2 in 1900 and it then fell steeply to
14.4 in 1933 except for a sharp increase after the end of the
First World War. The figure fell further in 1939 and rose
sharply again after the Second World War. By 1955 it had
fallen again to 15.0 but after this it began to rise again for an
undetermined reason. The figure is needed for planning such
services as maternity accommodation, schools, etc.

Mortality Statistics

Mortality statistics are based on information recorded when registration of death occurs. The causes of death are classified in accordance with the International Statistical Classification of Diseases, Injuries and Causes of Death without which international comparability would be almost impossible, but comparison of international death rates is still difficult. This is not only because of the differences in death certificates and in the way that causes of death are tabulated but also because there are differences in the proportions of deaths certified by qualified doctors, differences in the diagnostic facilities available and differences in the views on the relationships of one disease with another.

The *crude death rate* is the number of deaths per 1000 of the population. It is calculated by dividing the total number of deaths of people of all ages in one year by the estimated number of the population at the middle of the year and multiplying by 1000.

$$\text{Crude death rate per 1000 population} = \frac{\text{Total deaths, all ages}}{\text{Estimated population at June 30th}} \times 1000$$

The figure for 1969 was 11·8.

The death rate has little meaning on its own but is useful for making comparisons. For example the sex-age difference can be found by comparing one sex-age group with another or death rates of one year can be compared with another year, one area with another or one occupational group with another. Comparison of past and present death rates may establish a trend but changes in diagnosis will always affect these figures. As new diseases are discovered and more effective diagnostic methods used, patterns of mortality change but it does not necessarily mean that the disease in question is more lethal or widespread than before just simply that it is more easily recognized. Such changes cannot always be precisely estimated. Deaths from coronary artery disease and lung cancer seem to have increased enormously in recent years, particularly in men, but how much of this increase is due to the use of new terminology and how much to a real rise in the incidence of the two diseases is not known.

The *infant mortality rate* comprises deaths of all children under a year old and it is usually expressed as a rate per 1000 live births.

$$\text{Infant mortality rate} = \frac{\text{Deaths under 1 year of age in 1 year}}{\text{Live births in same year}} \times 1000$$

In 1969 the figure was 18·1. The infant mortality rate is specially important because of its close correlation with social conditions. The factors influencing any baby's progress are closely connected with the type of home in which he lives. If the living conditions are poor there is a much greater likelihood that the children may fall ill and that the outcome of that illness may be more serious. This will be reflected in the number of deaths of children under 1 year in that area. A deterioration in the social circumstances of any area, such as a sudden increase in the number of people unemployed, will rapidly be reflected in the infant mortality rate. Good paediatric services help in keeping the number of deaths down but living conditions are more important.

Separate periods within the first year are also usually defined. Deaths within the first four weeks are called *neonatal mortality*. About two thirds of the deaths in the first year occur during this period and the rate is higher in boys than in girls. In 1969 the figure was 11·4. Deaths over 4 weeks and under one year are called *post-neonatal mortality* and these are both expressed per 1000 live births as for the infant mortality rate.

A *stillbirth* is defined as being death of the fetus after the 28th week of pregnancy. The number of stillbirths and deaths during the first week of life are together known as the *perinatal morality rate* and this figure is expressed per 1000 total births, live and still. This figure indicates the hazards to the baby immediately before and after birth. Skilful midwifery may convert a likely stillbirth to a first week death but in either event the death will be shown in the perinatal mortality. In 1969 this was 23·4.

Maternal mortality rate includes deaths from maternal causes per 1000 total births (live and still) and is due to complications of pregnancy, abortion, delivery and the puerperium. It is related to standards of obstetric practice and the introduction of chemotherapy and antibiotics produced a dramatic fall as the dangers of death from puerperal infection were reduced. Later advances have lessened the hazards of toxaemia of pregnancy and of haemorrhage and have further reduced the maternal mortality rate.

Occupational mortality is analysed at the time of each census. Death registration includes the occupation of the deceased and the information is also on the census returns. Using these two pieces of information occupational death rates can be established. There are, however, some difficulties and limitations to be considered. There is often a variation in the information about a person's occupation as given by the head of the household at the census and by a near relative who registers the death. The last occupation is the one which is registered and this may not have been the usual occupation. More difficult is the fact that a job is often chosen because an individual feels he is physically suited to it; therefore mortality for a certain occupation may be low because only fit people apply and are accepted for it, or alternatively mortality may be high because another job is thought to be lighter and suitable for less robust people.

Morbidity Statistics

Morbidity statistics provide a picture of the amount of illness, disability and injury within a population but they must take account of several factors which do not have to be considered in mortality statistics. One illness may occur many times in the same person or he may have periods of remission during which he does not consider himself ill in the accepted sense; an illness may last varying lengths of time from a few hours to many years and it may be trivial or so serious that life is endangered. The amount of disturbance to his normal life pattern may also vary considerably. The figures are concerned with the number of people who are ill, the number of spells of illness that are experienced and the duration of these spells of illness. The figures are obtained from various official sources such as notifications of infectious diseases, certification of certain diseases for special benefits or allowances, records of road accidents and of industrial accidents and diseases. They are also compiled from hospital inpatient and outpatient records, general practitioners' clinical records, records kept by health and welfare centres and school medical records as well as by sickness surveys. The statistics are useful in many fields of work including the control of infectious disease, planning for the development of preventive and treatment services, estimating the economic importance of illness and its relation to social factors and for research into the cause and nature of disease and the efficiency of preventive and curative measures. The figures are, however, always somewhat inaccurate. Although many infectious diseases are notifiable the notifications are rarely complete, partly because of difficulty in diagnosis, and there are many minor infections such as influenza and the common cold which are not notifiable. Noninfectious disease ·is not notifiable and figures obtained from mortality statistics give a false impression because of the high mortality rate of some diseases and the low mortality rate of others.

Social Classes

Extensive use is made of a system of classification of occupations into five social classes depending on the general standing within the community of the occupations concerned. Social Class I is professional and includes such occupations as lawyers, doctors, clergymen, bank managers and company directors. Social Class II is called intermediate and includes farmers, managers, teachers, nurses and local government officers. Social Class III includes skilled workers such as fitters, clerks, engine drivers, miners, shop assistants and typists. Partly skilled workers such as farmworkers and machine minders are in Social Class IV, while Social Class V includes unskilled labourers of all kinds. The use of these classifications is mainly for comparison. The figures show, for example, an increasing gradient of mortality from Social Class I to Social Class V for some causes of death such as respiratory tuberculosis and bronchitis, while for diseases such as acute poliomyelitis and coronary artery disease the gradient is just as steep in the opposite direction. Infant mortality has always been lower in Social Class I and higher in Social Class V. Following the 1961 census 17 new socioeconomic groups were introduced. The aim was that each group should contain people of similar social, cultural and recreational standards.

14

Health Hazards

The development of the personal health services was dependent on the many medical discoveries that were made during the nineteenth century. In particular the discovery of pathogenic bacteria by Koch and the development of anti-septic techniques in surgery by Lister were significant. Among those advances which were particularly beneficial in the field of prevention of infectious disease was the development of the techniques of immunization.

The study of the characteristics of diseases which affect groups of people is called *epidemiology*. The discovery of the origin of a disease and of the way in which it spreads will give the key to its control. A close study is made of the *personal characteristics* common to all those people affected by a specific disease, including such things as diet, occupation and personal habits. The *time of onset* of a disease may be significant because of its relationship to changes of such factors as environment or habit. Another significant factor may be the *geographical distribution* of the disease.

Prevention of Infectious Diseases

The prevention of infectious disease usually demands that the spread of the disease from one person to another is interrupted in some way. In order to do this it is necessary to know the cause of the disease and the way in which it is spread.

Terms which are commonly used to describe transmissible diseases must be understood. A disease is *endemic* if it occurs constantly in any area; measles and chicken pox are endemic in Britain. If many cases of the same disease occur simultaneously an *epidemic* is occurring and if a series of epidemics spreads throughout the world it is known as a *pandemic*. *Sporadic* cases are those which have no connection between them.

The *incubation* period of a disease is the latent period between the infection and the first signs or symptoms of the disease. Knowledge of the likely length of this period is important in tracing the disease process as the incubation period may vary from a few hours (staphylococcal food poisoning) to weeks or months (syphilis, infective hepatitis).

Spread of Disease

The more serious infectious diseases are *notifiable* to the local authorities so that steps may be taken to trace the disease and prevent its spread. Examples of notifiable diseases are measles, whooping cough, tuberculosis, meningitis, poliomyelitis, tetanus and food poisoning. There are many others.

All serious infectious disease should be thoroughly investigated to find the cause and the factors which contribute to its spread. In this way it may be possible to prevent further cases occurring. People with whom the patient has been in contact and links with any other similar case should be investigated. If the disease is one not usually present in this country, such as smallpox, it is important to establish if contact has been made with someone who has recently been abroad. In gastrointestinal infections, which are often the result of eating contaminated food, a complete record is made of all food eaten during the likely incubation period.

Human Carriers

People may be infected with an organism and be the cause of infection in other people, without themselves having any symptoms. Such people are known as *carriers*. They may have recently had the disease and are still excreting the causative organism even though they seem to be better. They are known as convalescent carriers and such a condition is fairly common, and usually temporary, following diphtheria, typhoid, dysentery, poliomyelitis and streptococcal infections. Occasionally, the carrier state may be permanent, in which case the affected person may excrete the organism intermittently throughout his life. Typhoid fever is a disease which may give rise to the chronic carrier state.

Symptomless carriers may be totally unaware that they have ever had the disease but will nevertheless continue to excrete the organism following what was probably a subclinical attack. Salmonella infections, dysentery and poliomyelitis are examples of diseases which may give rise to such a state.

Environmental Influences on Disease

The properties of the **infecting organism** may influence the development of disease. If the patient is in contact with a particularly virulent organism he is more likely to contract the disease than with a less infective agent. Similarly the size of the infecting dose will affect the likelihood of developing or resisting the disease. The sudden emergence of a new strain of an organism, against which no resistance has been built up by a population, can be an important factor in producing an epidemic. Outbreaks of influenza in recent years which have spread across the world have been caused in this way.

The susceptibility of the **host** is a factor in the balance of natural forces which determines the incidence of disease. It depends on an individual's resistance to disease which may be lowered by local factors such as injury or cold or by general factors such as the state of health. The outcome may be development of the disease, development of a subclinical attack which may be followed by the symptomless carrier state or the individual may escape infection entirely.

The *environment* may affect either the organism or the host and the ease of spread will depend on it. In the winter months airborne infections such as colds and influenza are more common because cold weather encourages overcrowding in homes. Gastrointestinal diseases are more common in summer when warm weather assists bacterial multiplication in food and when flies are more common. Bad housing, overcrowded conditions and inadequate ventilation will assist the spread of many infectious diseases.

Personal Prevention

Much has been said in previous chapters about the contribution which can be made by each individual towards the maintenance of his own health which will play a considerable part in preventing infectious disease. Children must be taught to cover the nose and mouth with a handkerchief when sneezing or coughing. Paper handkerchiefs should be used by anyone who has influenza or a cold and after use they should be put into a bag so that they can be burnt. If linen handkerchiefs are used they should be soaked in disinfectant before being included in the family wash.

Gastrointestinal infections are very easily spread unless precautions are taken. In most instances the handle of the cistern and the door handle of the lavatory must be touched before the hands can be washed; the ideal situation is one in which the handbasin is situated in the same room as the lavatory. Lavatory seats should be of a washable plastic material and not of varnished wood. When the varnish wears off the wood becomes a trap for dirt, contamination and infection.

Animals

Many diseases can be transmitted to man through contact with animals. Mention has already been made of brucellosis which can be transmitted in infected milk; ornithosis, toxoplasmosis and infestation are other examples of diseases carried by animals. Where a pet is kept all crockery used for feeding the animal and the knives used for cutting up meat must be kept separate. Pets should not be allowed in bedrooms and children should be taught not to kiss animals, and to wash the hands after fondling or playing with them. If the pet becomes ill it should be isolated until it is better or has been seen by the vet.

Tropics

Insectborne diseases are not common in Britain, but brief mention should be made of malaria and plague.

Malaria, caused by *Plasmodium vivax*, is spread by the bite of an infected female anopheles mosquito, which is necessary for the completion of the life cycle of the malarial parasite. In order to prevent the disease the mosquitoes must be destroyed and the World Health Organization has mounted large scale campaigns to restrict breeding grounds by draining stagnant water and marshy areas. The widespread use of DDT and insect repellants is also helpful and the spraying of bedrooms before going to bed. Where the disease is highly epidemic the regular use of suppressive drugs is necessary and prompt treatment if the disease develops. Aircraft leaving an epidemic area must be sprayed before take-off so that infected insects are not transported to other areas.

Plague, caused by *Pasteurella pestis*, is endemic in Asia, India, South America and Central Africa and is transmitted to man by the bite of the rat flea. Widespread measures are taken in Britain to prevent infected rats from leaving ships in port. All ships are fumigated regularly to destroy the rats and every ship which berths must be 'ratproofed' to prevent rats leaving the ship.

Prevention of Non-infectious Disease

This is more involved than the prevention of transmissible diseases because each group of diseases must be studied separately. *Retrospective studies* depend on endeavouring to find common factors in the past history of a number of patients who are now suffering from a known disease. *Prospective studies* involve asking a large sample of people, who are apparently well, about their personal habits. Follow-up studies over a long period will reveal which of them, if any, develop certain diseases and what factors they have in common which may be implicated in the cause.

The greatest barrier to the prevention of non-infectious disease is that in many cases little is known about the cause. A study of the alterations in the incidence and severity of the disease over the years will give some valuable information; comparison of the disease as it occurs in different levels of the same community, in different areas of the same country and in different countries may indicate the cause. Other factors of interest are the seasonal variations, the effects of heredity or race, the differences in sex and personality, the social factors and the mortality, all of which may help in defining the cause.

Cancer

Some diseases can be prevented but in many cases the disease is not recognized until it has developed and the preventive aspects are confined to preventing deterioration and complications. Prevention of cancer may be helped by recognizing a precancerous condition and removing it before it spreads, as in cancer of the cervix.

Women over the age of 25 years should have a routine test performed regularly at three- to five-year intervals. Removal and examination of moisture and cells from the vagina may reveal a precancerous condition which can then be treated. Removal of the irritating precipitating factor, such as cigarette smoking in cancer of the lung, may also help. A study of the increased incidence of cancer of the lung in recent years brought to light its connection with smoking.

Cancer of the breast is common in women and some authorities recommend self-examination of the breasts at regular intervals to detect the presence of a lump. This should be carried out after a menstrual period or, following the menopause, on a predetermined day, the first day of the month for example.

Recent studies of the incidence of certain types of cancer has revealed such facts as the higher incidence of cancer of the mouth and pharynx in Ireland, but a correspondingly low incidence of cancer of the lung and cervix. Japan has a relatively low incidence of cancer of the lung and breast but a higher incidence of cancer of the stomach, but if Japanese people emigrate to the USA the incidence quickly approximates to that of their new country. Studies by Social Class reveal that carcinoma of the lung and stomach is lowest in Social Class I and highest in Social Class V – but the trend is reversed in the incidence of leukaemia.

Coronory Thrombosis

The success of preventive measures against coronary thrombosis have been equivocal. Because a high blood cholesterol level has been a common finding, regular tests have been carried out and those who had a high level of cholesterol have been given a diet which is low in animal fat, encouraged to avoid obesity and smoking and to take regular exercise. Unfortunately statistics do not show that these measures have had any marked success.

Chronic Bronchitis

Chronic bronchitis can be helped by abstinence from cigarette smoking and by reduction of air pollution, both of which are difficult to enforce.

Mental Health

Much has been said in earlier chapters about the maintenance of mental health. Hereditary, developmental, domestic, occupational and environmental factors all play an important part in the prevention of mental illness and the early recognition of emotional instability may help to prevent serious breakdown at a later date.

Early Detection of Disease

At the present time there is little in the way of routine medical checks in this country, though it is fairly common in countries such as the USA and Russia. The occasional surveys which have been carried out have revealed considerable undiagnosed disease; and example is the Bedford survey which uncovered 356 cases of asymptomatic diabetes in a population of 65 000.

Mass radiography has been responsible for the discovery of a considerable number of cases of various types of chest disease. Campaigns are often launched by local authorities to encourage people to check their eyesight or hearing. Most people will go to their doctors if they feel unwell or have pain. Loss of vision, severe pain in the eye, progressive weight loss, persistent alteration in the pattern of bowel habits, loss of blood from any part of the body and any lumps, swellings or persistent pain are symptoms which indicate that a medical check-up is a matter of necessity.

Noise

Noise is a contributory factor in the creation of nervous tension but little is done actively to combat it. Some people are able to tolerate noise more easily than others but there is evidence to show that people who have what appears to be a high noise tolerance are expending a great deal of energy to insulate themselves against it and this in itself increases nervous tension.

In industry noisy processes create many problems. Efficiency falls because excessive noise increases industrial fatigue, though the rate at which efficiency declines will depend on the noise tolerance of each individual. Continuous loud noise such as occurs in riveting and boiler making will eventually result in a loss of hearing which may be permanent, while repetitive sounds lead to increased irritability. Ear muffs or ear plugs should be used by workers in a noisy environment, or in some cases special walls are erected to screen noisy machines. Less noisy machines have been developed but these are expensive.

In areas where noise is a problem all employees should have their hearing tested before employment and at regular intervals of two years while a worker who complains of auditory symptoms should be suspended from noisy tasks.

Irradiation

Ionizing radiations are present in small amounts in the environment. This background irradiation comes partly from the sun, partly from the soil, from manufactured items such as bricks and from the human body. Radioactive carbon which is present in skeletons has enabled archaeologists to estimate the dates of discoveries they make.

There are just measurable amounts of radioactive substances in cereals and other foods. Strontium is present in plants which are grazed by cattle and it is secreted in milk and finds its way into human bone tissue. The same concentration has been defined and the level in Britain is very low and decreasing.

People whose work brings them into contact with radiation, such as radiologists, are at a greater risk and special precautions must be taken to safeguard their health. Patients treated by radiotherapy are also a special group. There is evidence that among such people there is a higher incidence of chronic myeloid leukaemia due to excessive radiation and this is also true of survivors of the atomic bomb attacks on Nagasaki and Hiroshima. Radiation affects cells most when they are reproducing, first inhibiting the process, then increasing it. Larger doses cause the cells to lose their reproductive powers entirely. This is particularly serious when the reproductive organs are affected as sterility may result, or a less damaging dose may cause congenital malformations in children. There is some evidence that children of mothers who are X-rayed during early pregnancy may have a higher incidence of leukaemia.

The International Commission on Radiation Protection in liaison with the World Health Organization make recommendations for protective measures against excessive radiation. Distance and shielding are the main protective measures. X-ray rooms and equipment are shielded and workers must wear protective clothing.

Lead

Lead can be taken into the system by inhalation and by ingestion and it has been the cause of occupational disease in miners and smelters, car workers, sheet metal workers and spray painters among others. Chronic lead poisoning is not uncommon in young children aged between one to three years who readily develop raised lead blood levels and may suffer brain damage if not treated. Mention has already been made of 'pica', the habit of eating unusual substances, but poisoning may also occur in children who live near the sites of major road works or where lead is being used as an additive to petrol.

Lead is present in varying amounts in soil, water, food and air and the major source of intake in humans is from food. It accumulates in the bones where it replaces calcium. Continual efforts are being made to reduce pollution of the environment by lead substances.

15

The Effect of Immigration on Health

In this context the word 'immigrant' means anyone who has come as a settler into another country and who has therefore to make both biological and psychological adjustments in order to fit into the new community.

Housing

All new arrivals to any country must find a job and a place to live. Living accommodation is frequently shared with friends or relations and may mean overcrowding and inadequate communal facilities. Where there is multiple occupancy there tends to be more rubbish but rarely extra collections so garbage may accumulate and attract flies and vermin. The wiring and plumbing are also overstrained and may not function adequately. All these factors are likely to affect the health of the newcomers.

Infection and Immunity

The arrival in any country of numbers of immigrants alters the reservoir of infection in the host country. The immigrants may bring with them a strain of disease to which the hosts have little or no immunity or the immigrants may fall victim to an infection to which they have low immunity. In either case the overall incidence of disease is increased and therefore the likelihood of spread is greater. The amount of infection passing between the two communities will depend on the degree of integration, which may be restricted to begin with though it will increase as time goes by.

The degree of natural immunity to infection is often less in immigrant children and it is thought this may be due in part to an inadequate intake of protein during the early years. In many countries meat is very expensive and protein intake may be largely from cereals; on arrival in the host country the familiar foods are not available and mothers may be reluctant to try new ones and so the nutrition of the child is worse than it was before immigration.

Cultural Differences and Adaptation

The arrival of large numbers of immigrants alters the sex-age distribution in the host country. Frequently the young married men arrive first followed soon after by their wives and families. There are initially few young children and few very elderly people. A few years after arrival there will be many more very young children.

The new arrivals have to adapt immunologically, culturally and sometimes linguistically to a new situation. The environment is likely to be very different and the changes needed have to be made very quickly in many cases so that there will be considerably more stress in daily living than is found among the indigenous population. This may result in increased ill health.

It is necessary to be aware of cultural differences so that these can be accepted as differences of custom rather than as differences of moral behaviour. At the same time unless this knowledge is sound, abnormal behaviour may be accepted as simply being unfamiliar when it may be in fact the first sign of overwhelming stress.

Where a large number of immigrants from one country settle close together in the new country they give much mutual support and the amount of mental illness which occurs does not appear to be exceptionally high. In many cases however the children face greater problems as they try to fit into the life of the host country at school and to family life after school which may have changed little from the life they knew before immigration. In addition there may be a new language to learn, or at least colloquialisms, and it is not uncommon to hear children speaking two distinct types of English, varying according to the person to whom they are speaking.

Religion

Religious customs vary considerably and an understanding of them is important as they may affect the health of the individual both directly and indirectly.

Nearly all Pakistanis are Moslem and as such are forbidden to eat pork. There are also regulations concerning the way in which any animal providing meat must be slaughtered. During the month of Ramadan no food or drink is taken between dawn and dusk and although people who are ill are not required to fast in this way many may want to and the spiritual achievement may be more beneficial than persuading an ardent Moslem not to fast.

Among newly arrived Moslem immigrants the custom of Purdah may prevent women from leaving home to attend clinics or the doctor and may even prevent a mother from calling the doctor if a child is ill. Delay until the man of the house or a male relative comes home from work may be disastrous when a small child is ill.

Of the Indian population 90 per cent are Hindu and as the cow is considered a sacred animal beef will not be eaten by a Hindu. Some Hindus will not eat any meat and may even refuse eggs, though milk is usually acceptable. Such a diet may be lacking in protein unless vegetable proteins such as pulses, wholemeal flour and oatmeal are included in the diet in sufficient quantity.

Sikhs are part of a reformed movement within Hinduism and many are from the region of the Punjab. A Sikh will not eat beef but will eat other meats. The word Singh is a title which is used to denote a male Sikh, just as Kaur denotes a female Sikh. Immigrants who are unfamiliar with the Western custom of using a forename (or Christian name) followed by a family name (or surname) must be persuaded to use a family name and to stick to it.

Clothing and Warmth

Those immigrants who come from warm climates will need advice about the provision of warm clothing in winter months for school children and babies as well as for themselves. Equally an overclothed baby in an overheated room is at risk. Where the new arrivals settle in an area already inhabited by their own countrymen advice is freely given and well accepted. The problem is greater where the settling family is isolated and reluctant to become integrated.

Advice will also be needed about the most effective way to heat the house. Paraffin heaters and open fires are both dangerous where there are children, or adults wearing flowing clothes such as saris and all such fires must be adequately guarded.

Food

It is not uncommon to find low haemoglobin levels in newly arrived immigrant babies. Many have been breast fed for longer than is customary in the West and have used up the iron stored in the liver which may itself have been inadequate because of the poorer nutritional state of the mother. Together with the later age at which iron-containing foods are introduced into the diet this often produces a fairly severe degree of iron-deficiency anaemia.

Older children who are not vegetarian often receive a better standard of diet after arrival than they have been used to. They tend to eat more meat and other protein foods and may eat more fruit. The child who is a vegetarian is less well off because the variety of food that he has been used to is not available. In Britain it is necessary for infants to have supplementary vitamin D in their food and immigrant mothers may be unaware of this problem. In addition the synthesis of vitamin D by the action of sunlight on skin will be reduced in dark-skinned children because of the screening effect of the melanin pigment in the skin.

Background Readings

Montague, A. (1964) *Life Before Birth*, Harlow: Longmans.

Parr, J. A. & Young, R. A. (1966) *Health, Happiness and Survival*, London: Heinemann.

Emery, A. (1971) *Elements of Medical Genetics*, Edinburgh: Churchill Livingstone.

Millar, S. (1971) *Psychology of Play*, Harmondsworth: Penguin.

Bowlby, J. & Fry, M. (1970) *Child Care and the Growth of Love*, Harmondsworth: Penguin.

Illingworth, R. S. (1968) *Normal Child*, Edinburgh: Churchill Livingstone.

Jelliffe, D. B. (1968) *Child Health in the Tropics*, London: Edward Arnold.

Sheridan, M. (1960) *Developmental Progress of Infants and Young Children*, London: HMSO.

DHSS (1972) *Immunization against Infectious Diseases*, London: HMSO.

Newson, J. & Newson, E. (1971) *Patterns of Infant Care in an Urban Community*, Harmondsworth: Penguin.

Family Welfare Association (1972) *Guide to the Social Services*, London: Macdonald & Evans.

Meredith Davies, J. B. (1971) *Preventive Medicine, Community Health and Social Services*, London: Baillière Tindall.

Davis, K. (1970) *Human Society*, London: Collier Macmillan.

Fromm, E. (1942) *Fear of Freedom*, London: Routledge & Kegan Paul.

Edge, P. (1971) *Child Care and Management*, London: Faber & Faber.

Valentine, C. W. (1956) *Normal Child and some of his Abnormalities*, Harmondsworth: Penguin.

Hadfield, J. A. (1970) *Childhood and Adolescence*, Harmondsworth: Penguin.

Illingworth, R. S. (1964) *The Normal Schoolchild*, London: Heinemann.

Lee, C. (1969) *Growth and Development of Children*, Harlow: Longmans.

Turner, M. (1965) *Faulty Posture – its effects and treatment*, Harlow: Longmans.

Sutherland, J. D. (1971) *Towards Community Mental Health*, London: Tavistock.

Laurence, D. R. (1966) *Clinical Pharmacology*, Edinburgh: Churchill Livingstone.

Swinson, A. (1965) *Casebook of Medical Detection*, London: Davies.

Glatt, M. M., Pittman, Gillespie, Hills. (1967) *The Drug Scene in Great Britain*, London: Edward Arnold.

Royal College of Physicians (1971) *Smoking and Health Now*, London: Pitman Medical.

Caruana, S. & Scowen, P. (ed.) (1973) *Alcohol and Alcoholism*, London: Edsall & Co. Ltd.

Gunn, A. (1970) *The Privileged Adolescent*, Medical & Technical Publishing Co.

Fleming, C. M. (1967) *Adolescence – its Social Psychology*, London: Routledge & Kegan Paul.

Mead, M. (1970) *Growing Up in New Guinea*, Harmondsworth: Penguin.

Mead, M. (1970) *Coming of Age in Samoa*, Harmondsworth: Penguin.

Mussen, P. (1964) *The Psychological Development of the Child*, Hemel Hempstead: Prentice Hall.

Ffrench, G. *Occupational Health*, Medical & Technical Publishing Co.

Craddock, D. (1969) *Obesity and its Management*, Edinburgh: Churchill Livingstone.

Malleson, J. (1949) *Change of Life*, Harmondsworth: Penguin.

Yudkin, J. (1970) *This Slimming Business*, Harmondsworth: Penguin.

Irvine, R. E., Bagnall, M. K. & Smith, B. J. (1970) *The Older Patient*, London: E.U.P.

Rudd, T. N. (1967) *Human Relations in Old Age*, London: Faber & Faber.

Kemp, R. (1965) *New Look at Geriatrics*, London: Pitman Medical.

Francis, G. (1973) *Caring for the Elderly*, London: Heinemann.

Sutton, M. (1966) *Cancer Explained*, London: Evans.

Waldbolt, G. L. (1973) *Health Effects of Environmental Pollutants*, London: Kimpton (Henry) Publishers.

Dodge, J. S. (1969) *The Field Worker in Immigrant Health*, Staples Press.

General Books

Blindness

Lunt, L. (1965) *If you make a noise I can't see*, Connecticut: Verry.

Blackhall, D. S. (1962) *This House had Windows*, New York: Astor-Honor.

Maladjustment

Axline, V. M. (1969) *Dibs: in search of self*, New York: Ballantine.

Difficulty with Words

Browning, E. (1973) *I can't see what you're saying*, New York: Coward-McCann.

Critchley, M. (1972) *The Dyslexic Child*, Springfield: C. C. Thomas.

Autism

Park, C. C. (1972) *The Seige: The First Eight Years of an Autistic Child*, Little.

Educational Subnormality

Wilson, L. (1971) *This Stranger, My Son*, London: Hutchinsons.

Hunt, N. (1967) *The World of Nigel Hunt: The Diary of a Mongoloid Youth*, New York: Garrett-Helix.

Physical Handicap

Wilson, D. C. (1971) *Handicap Race: The Inspiring Story of Roger Arnett*, Maidenhead: McGraw-Hill.

Opie, J. (1957) *Over My Dead Body*, New York: Dutton.

Wilson, D. C. (1971) *Hilary: The Brave World of Hilary Pole*, Maidenhead: McGraw-Hill.

Index

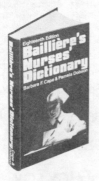
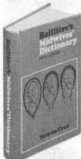
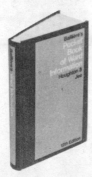

THE NURSES AIDS SERIES NAS

The Nurses' Aids Series is planned to meet the needs of the student nurse during training, and later in qualifying for another part of the Register, by providing a set of textbooks covering most of the subjects included in the general part of the Register and certain specialist subjects. The pupil nurse, too, will find many of these books of particular value and help in practical bedside training. The Series conforms to three factors important to the student:

1. All the authors are nurses who know exactly what the student requires.

ANAESTHETICS FOR NURSES
1971 • 1st edn. • £1.10

ANATOMY AND PHYSIOLOGY FOR NURSES*
1972 • 8th edn. • Limp £1.20 • Hard £2.00

ARITHMETIC IN NURSING
1972 • 4th edn. • Limp £1.10 • Hard £2.00

EAR, NOSE AND THROAT NURSING
1972 • 5th edn. • Limp £1.10 • Hard £2.00

MEDICAL NURSING
1972 • 8th edn. • Limp £1.20 • Hard £2.00

MICROBIOLOGY FOR NURSES*
1972 • 4th edn. • Limp £1.00 • Hard £1.50

OBSTETRIC AND GYNAECOLOGICAL NURSING*
1969 • 1st edn. • Limp £1.20 • Hard £2.00

ORTHOPAEDICS FOR NURSES*
1971 • 4th edn. • Limp £1.20 • Hard £2.00

PAEDIATRIC NURSING
1974 • 4th edn. • Limp £1.30 • Hard £2.00

OPHTHALMOLOGY FOR NURSES
1975 • 1st edn. • Limp £1.20 • Hard £2.00

THE NURSES' AIDS SERIES ∏∏S

2. The books are frequently revised to ensure that advances in knowledge reach the student as soon as practicable.

3. The Aids are well printed and easy to read, clearly illustrated, and modestly priced.

Thus this famous Series, which covers all aspects of nursing studies — scientific, theoretical and practical — contributes significantly to nurse training in this country and abroad.

PERSONAL AND COMMUNITY HEALTH
1969 • 2nd edn. • Limp 80p • Hard £2.00

PHARMACOLOGY FOR NURSES
1975 • 4th edn. • Limp £1.20 • Hard £2.00

PRACTICAL NURSING*
1971 • 11th edn. • Limp £1.10 • Hard £2.00

PRACTICAL PROCEDURES FOR NURSES
1969 • 1st edn. • £1.10

PSYCHIATRIC NURSING
1973 • 4th edn. • Limp £1.10 • Hard £2.00

PSYCHOLOGY FOR NURSES
1975 • 4th edn. • Limp £1.20 • Hard £2.00

SURGICAL NURSING*
9th edn. • Limp £1.20 • Hard £2.00

THEATRE TECHNIQUE
1967 • 4th edn. • £1.10

TROPICAL HYGIENE AND NURSING* *New edition in preparation.*

DO-IT-YOURSELF
REVISION FOR NURSES
BOOKS 1, 2, 3, 4, 5 & 6

E. J. HULL and B. J. ISAACS

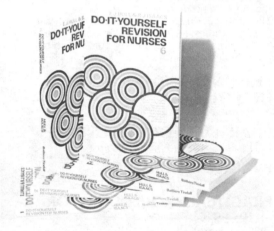

The six books of this series provide a comprehensive framework for revision of the GNC syllabus and developments made since to it. The student reviews a subject of choice, answers questions selected from recent State Final Examinations, and marks her replies against the model answers provided.

'Highly recommended to all student nurses as a planned guide to revision.' *Nursing Times*

'ZRN Finalists and aspiring ZENs would benefit enormously were they to use these little books as intended…Tutors will have cause to be grateful, students even more so.' *Zambia Nurse*

1970-1972 • **Books 1-6** • *135 pp average •
illustrated • Books 1, 2, 3 & 4—70p each •
Books 5 & 6—60p each*

STANDARD TEXTBOOKS

PERRY/WARD ADMINISTRATION & TEACHING

"This is a book which has long been needed. Every trained nurse could learn something from it. While ward sisters put into practice the ideals and ideas outlined, we need have no fears for 'patient care' in our hospitals nor for the practical training of the nurse."
Nursing Mirror £2.50

BURR/SWIRE'S HANDBOOK OF PRACTICAL NURSING

This is a well-known textbook for the practical nurse, accurate and written in a clear, easy-to-read style.
6th edn. £1.10

MEERING & STACEY/NURSERY NURSING — A HANDBOOK FOR NURSERY NURSES

"This book is written in a clear and simple style emphasizing the relationship between the emotional, intellectual and physical growth during infancy and childhood...a valuable reference book for all nurses interested in nursery work..." *The Lamp*
5th edn. £2.75

ELLIOTT & RYZ/VENEREAL DISEASES: TREATMENT & NURSING

'Containing concise, factual and up-to-date information on the symptoms, signs, treatment and nursing management of patients with venereal diseases, it is eminently suitable for nurses both in training and those who have completed training.'
Queen's Nursing Journal £1.80

HUTTON/BASIC NURSING CARE
A Guide for Nursing Auxiliaries

A practical, induction period, reference book for nursing auxiliaries in association with in-service training schemes and ward procedure manuals. *80p*

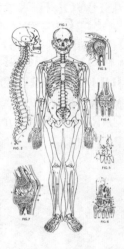